Mind Race

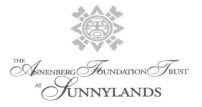

THE

ANNENBERG FOUNDATION TRUST
AT SUNNYLANDS

The Annenberg Foundation Trust at Sunnylands'
Adolescent Mental Health Initiative

Patrick Jamieson, Ph.D., *series editor*

In addition to *Mind Race,* other books in this series for
young people are planned on the following topics:

Depression (2006)
Addiction (2007)
Eating Disorders (2007)
Obsessive-Compulsive Disorder (2007)
Schizophrenia (2007)
Social Anxiety Disorder (2007)

Also available in the series for parents and other adults:

*If Your Adolescent Has Depression
or Bipolar Disorder (2005)*
Dwight L. Evans, M.D., and Linda Wasmer Andrews

If Your Adolescent Has an Eating Disorder (2005)
B. Timothy Walsh, M.D., and V. L. Cameron

If Your Adolescent Has an Anxiety Disorder (2006)
Edna B. Foa, Ph.D., and Linda Wasmer Andrews

If Your Adolescent Has Schizophrenia (2006)
Raquel E. Gur, M.D., Ph.D., and Ann Braden Johnson, Ph.D.

Mind Race

*A Firsthand Account of
One Teenager's Experience
with Bipolar Disorder*

Patrick E. Jamieson, Ph.D.
with Moira A. Rynn, M.D.

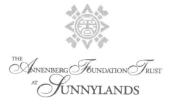

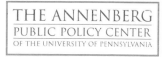

The Annenberg Foundation Trust at Sunnylands'
Adolescent Mental Health Initiative

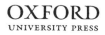

OXFORD
UNIVERSITY PRESS

2006

OXFORD

UNIVERSITY PRESS

Oxford University Press, Inc., publishes works that
further Oxford University's objective of excellence
in research, scholarship, and education.

The Annenberg Foundation Trust at Sunnylands
The Annenberg Public Policy Center of the University of Pennsylvania
Oxford University Press

Oxford   New York
Auckland   Cape Town   Dar es Salaam   Hong Kong   Karachi
Kuala Lumpur   Madrid   Melbourne   Mexico City   Nairobi
New Delhi   Shanghai   Taipei   Toronto

With offices in
Argentina   Austria   Brazil   Chile   Czech Republic   France   Greece
Guatemala   Hungary   Italy   Japan   Poland   Portugal   Singapore
South Korea   Switzerland   Thailand   Turkey   Ukraine   Vietnam

Copyright © 2006 by Patrick E. Jamieson

Published by Oxford University Press, Inc.
198 Madison Avenue, New York, New York 10016
www.oup.com

Oxford is a registered trademark of Oxford University Press

Library of Congress Cataloging-in-Publication Data
Jamieson, Patrick E., 1973–
Mind race : A Firsthand Account of One Teenager's Experience
With Bipolar Disorder/ Patrick E. Jamieson with
Moira A. Rynn.
    p. cm. — (Adolescent mental health initiative)
"The Annenberg Foundation Trust at Sunnylands, the Annenberg Public
Policy Center."
Includes bibliographical references and index.
ISBN-13: 978-0-19-530906-5 (cloth-13)   ISBN-10: 0-19-530906-5 (cloth)
ISBN-13: 978-0-19-530905-8 (paper-13)   ISBN-10: 0-19-530905-7 (pbk)
1. Manic-depressive illness in adolescence.
I. Rynn, Moira A. II. Title. III. Series.
RC516.J35 2006   616.89'5—dc22   2006002139

Parts of the Diagnostic Criteria for Manic Episode and for Major Depressive Episode are
reprinted with permission from *The Diagnostic and Statistical Manual of Mental Disorders*,
Fourth Edition, Text Revision. Copyright © 2000, American Psychiatric Association.

9 8 7 6 5 4 3 2 1
Printed in the United States of America
on acid-free paper

For my son, Finnian James

Contents

Foreword

The Adolescent Mental Health Initiative (AMHI) was created by The Annenberg Foundation Trust at Sunnylands to share with mental health professionals, parents, and adolescents the advances in treatment and prevention now available to adolescents with mental health disorders. The Initiative was made possible by the generosity and vision of Ambassadors Walter and Leonore Annenberg, and the project was administered through the Annenberg Public Policy Center of the University of Pennsylvania in partnership with Oxford University Press.

The Initiative began in 2003 with the convening, in Philadelphia and New York, of seven scholarly commissions made up of over 150 leading psychiatrists and psychologists from around the country. Chaired by Drs. Edna B. Foa, Dwight L. Evans, B. Timothy Walsh, Martin E.P. Seligman, Raquel E. Gur, Charles P. O'Brien, and Herbert Hendin, these commissions were tasked with assessing the state of scientific research on the prevalent mental disorders whose onset occurs predominantly between the ages of 10 and 22. Their collective findings now appear in a book for mental health professionals and policymakers titled *Treating and Preventing Adolescent Mental Health Disorders* (2005). As the first product of the Initiative, that book also identified a research agenda that would best advance our ability to prevent and treat these disorders, among them anxiety disorders, depression and bipolar disorder, eating disorders, substance abuse, and schizophrenia.

The second prong of the Initiative's three-part effort is a series of smaller books for general readers. Some of the books are designed primarily for parents of adolescents with a specific mental health disorder. And some, including this one, are aimed at adolescents themselves who are struggling with a mental illness. All of the books draw their scientific information in part from the AMHI professional volume, presenting it in a manner that is accessible to general readers of different ages. The "teen books" also feature the real-life story of one young person who has struggled with—and now manages—a given mental illness. They serve both as a source of solid research about the illness and as a roadmap to recovery for afflicted young people. Thus they offer a unique combination of medical science and firsthand practical wisdom in an effort to inspire adolescents to take an active role in their own recovery.

The third part of the Sunnylands Adolescent Mental Health Initiative consists of two websites. The first, www.CopeCare Deal.org, addresses teens. The second, www.oup.com/us/teenmentalhealth, provides updates to the medical community on matters discussed in *Treating and Preventing Adolescent Mental Health Disorders*, the AMHI professional book.

We hope that you find this volume, as one of the fruits of the Initiative, to be helpful and enlightening.

Patrick Jamieson, Ph.D., *Series Editor*
Adolescent Risk Communication Institute
Annenberg Public Policy Center
University of Pennsylvania
Philadelphia, PA

Preface

Having bipolar disorder, or manic depression as it is also called, doesn't have to be depressing. Manic and maniac are different words—different people.

Mind Race is the book I searched for and could not find when I learned at age 15 that there was a name for the exhilarating sense that I was fearlessly catapulting through the galaxy, gravity-free and giddy one moment—then suddenly terrified after a sleepless night and barely able to function during a mind-numbing low. The name was bipolar disorder: a lifelong but treatable condition.

The life of a person with bipolar disorder can be tumultuous. When I have been in the state of mania I've had thinking that I couldn't stop, lying in bed for hours with words bounding and rebounding between my ears, knowing that a night without sleep increased the likelihood of hospitalization. When depressed, I have trouble putting ideas together at all. I slow down dramatically and a minute seems like an hour. There is no pleasure, and I stop remembering my dreams.

This is a first-person account for adolescents and young adults faced with the diagnosis of bipolar disorder. It is also for their mothers, fathers, sisters, brothers, and friends. It is meant as a supplement rather than as a substitute for the excellent books that are now available on bipolar disorder (some of which are mentioned in the Resources section of this book). *Mind Race* is about the way life changes when, in addition to the usual hormonal havoc, an adolescent must navigate a chronic, mind-altering condition. It is written both to explain to young people how knowledge can help those with bipolar disorder and what treatments are available for it, and to provide advice on how to cope with its effects. I invite you to share my experiences.

Before you start reading, let me offer a few preliminary notes. First, I have changed the names of most of the people mentioned in the book's autobiographical chapters in order to protect their privacy, and in Chapter 5, I have condensed into one narrative the most meaningful experiences I had during six hospitalizations in a psychiatric ward. Also, although I discuss medication and other treatments, I am not recommending that you adopt the regimen that my doctors and I have developed for me. The best course of treatment for you should be determined in consultation with a qualified doctor, who will assess your symptoms and prescribe and monitor your medication and its effects, and a qualified therapist, who will help you come to terms with this disorder and the life adjustments it requires. Bipolar disorder is classified primarily into two categories—bipolar I and bipolar II—and the illness manifests itself differently from one person to another. The events described in this book surround my experiences with bipolar I, though you may find that your own experiences are quite different. Moreover, bipolar disorder can be complicated by what are called "comorbidities"—other disorders that occur at the same time. A person can have bipolar disorder and an eating disorder, or bipolar disorder and obsessive-compulsive disorder (a type of anxiety disorder), or bipolar disorder and many other combinations of mental illness, including substance abuse. What is important to keep in mind is that each person's experience of a mental illness is as unique as that person him- or herself. And so my own story is told here in part to encourage you to face your own unique circumstances, your own unique diagnosis, and to seek the professional help that is right for you.

Acknowledgments

I thank everyone who encouraged me over the many years and transformations *Mind Race* has taken, and apologize in advance to anyone who is left out. I thank my wife, Laura, for everything she does and my son, Finnian, to whom this book is dedicated, as well as my mom, dad, and brother Rob. I also thank the Annenbergs and the Annenberg Foundation Trust at Sunnylands; Dr. Dan Romer for the optimism; Dean Delli Carpini for the support; Eian More for making my life easier; Richard Cardona, who helps me stay sane; Karen Riley for the editorial assistance; Abby Zimmerman for helping to research this book; Kate Kenski for being such a good friend through graduate school; Dr. Jaroslav Pelikan for showing me what an academic and, more importantly, what a human being should be; Zach and Nick; Dr. Moira Rynn for acting as the medical adviser on this book, and Doctors Marvin Lazerson, Martin Seligman, and Dwight Evans for reviewing earlier drafts. I wouldn't be here without all the teachers who pushed me, especially the history and writing teachers who took a chance on a troubled kid. I am also grateful to this book's editors, Marion Osmun and Sarah Harrington from Oxford University Press.

P. E. J.
Philadelphia, PA

Mind Race

Chapter One

There and Back:
A Bipolar Trip

Mania is about desperately seeking to live life at a more passionate
level, taking second and sometimes third helpings on food, alcohol,
drugs, sex, and money, trying to live a whole life in one day.

—Andy Behrman, *Electroboy: A Memoir of Mania* (2002)

L et me try to show you the racing thoughts of my manic
mind:

IN THE GARDEN AND EATEN

Under the log, Pill bug, Maggot, grub,
Brook, stream, Fanciful dream, Bridge of stone; man named
    Malone.
Glistening, rushing, flowing, growing,
Moist, wet, and crowing.
Cradled in womb, a sloth's tomb,
Geese, sparrows, not—good-bed-fellows,
Youth taunting, haunting, Dark December. Remember.
Conjure sap. Conjure sun. Conjure lilies and lilacs. Conjure spring.
Floating freely, a loon, three-mile cocoon. Don't
Touch the ground. Rebound.
Milky sheets, wet heat, autumn shiver, Pray to the lord, deliver,
    forgive her.
Fast as lightning, frightening, an October to remember, wait for
    December! Halloween or Christmas, do not dismiss us. Ripples
    of Waves paved, craved. I rush the mountain and fall.
Through sycamores. Small. Stall.
Amber, tight-ribbed and slender, lumbering ax, tripped by rock,
    trapped by shock

Defrocked. Blue belles writhe.
Inside.
Hide.
Arms unwound. Deafening sounds. In borderless towns.
Head crowned. Drowned. Rebound.
King of the night.
Culling the shaft, right hand drawn fast, Jared the Carver.
Swing with delight, fright, snap back, sap slack, roots. Warm,
    solid, together, Grab the tool, Shank grafted in fiber,
2000 years inside her. Fire. I find her.

It isn't Dylan Thomas or even Jakob Dylan. I know that now, but when I wrote it early one morning in a wash of mania and alcohol, I thought this poem was brilliant. When born of a stable mind, these thoughts would be metaphors to me; when manic, I live them.

The playful, mind-expanding sense of euphoria that mania brings can last for moments, days, or weeks. If you haven't been there, all I have to offer are analogies. Remember the first time you thought you were in love, an emotion that seemed original, overpowering, and real. Life became anticipation and fulfillment all focused on one person. Anticipating spending time with her. Repeating, "She loves me!" Now imagine experiencing those feelings for your toaster, marveling at how the gears and coils work in perfect synchrony, admiring your reflection in its shiny surface. Your focus shifts to an orange. You marvel that the juice is captured in tiny cells. Nature is sharing her secrets with you.

Life feels like it is supercharged with possibility. You feel joyful about the prospect of going shopping later that day. You are talkative and feel bold, powerful, attractive, charming, and cunning—all at the same time. Ordinary activities are extraordinary! Supermarkets are temples with altars stacked with cereals and pastries, puddings and peanuts, milk and mayonnaise—everything you could eat or cook or paint or dance to. My manic world is alliterative and filled with rhymes and puns: "Through sycamores. Small. Stall. . . . Fire. I find her."

I become the Energizer Bunny on a supercharger. "Why does everybody else need so much sleep?" I wonder. I hastily finish next week's homework and write poetry late into the night. Hours pass like minutes, minutes like seconds. If I sleep, it is briefly and I awake refreshed, thinking, "This is going to be the best day of my life!"

Bipolar High School

The next day the words don't flow; they gush. The only thing keeping pace with my mind is the phone bill as I reconnect to a galaxy of friends and acquaintances. The day after a late-night, hour-long call, one of my friends eyes me quizzically. Observing my newfound buoyancy, my favorite teacher asks if I'm all right. My baseball coach reams me out for trying to steal third without waiting for the sign. I blow him off. Though I failed to make the base, the mad dash freed me from growing tendrils on second.

"Why does everybody drive so slowly?" I wonder. "And walk so slowly and talk so slowly and think so slowly? If they don't start living soon, they will all mold."

When manic, I am more confident, more irritable, and more verbally aggressive. My thoughts bombard me from every direction. When manic, I am happy when alone and happier when others are attracted to my energy.

When manic, I am happy when alone and happier when others are attracted to my energy.

During a manic state I can stay up all of one night and get by on a few hours of sleep the next before crashing into a longer sleep. I remember my brother pulling off my shoes without untying the laces (you expect more from an older brother?). He had arrived home from the university one afternoon and found me still asleep. When the hours normally spent awake and asleep lose their distinctiveness, one can wake up not knowing if it is A.M. or P.M.

In one of the ironies of the illness, manic exuberance is a prelude—not an end state. It's great for a time, but it doesn't last. What follows isn't worth the exhilaration of the earlier euphoria. My mania is a mountain from which I abruptly plunge into depression or from which I ascend into an even higher summit of mania, where playfulness becomes verbal aggression and fanciful exchanges with family and friends become monologues. I think I know more than other people when manic; consequently I drive words like knives into friend and family alike.

Before, sleeplessness was a blessing; it is now a curse. Where just moments before, it was leaping and frolicking harmlessly, my mind now races dangerously. It is the driver; I am the engine. I don't control the ignition or the accelerator. I live a wakeful nightmare of fantasies into which I incorporate the people who try to enter my world. They are no longer benign presences charmed by my cleverness. They are trying to trick or injure me. I summon emotions that I don't ordinarily feel to slice and dice these adversaries like a Vegematic.

After several weeks my mania ends as I descend into a world of muted sounds and gray shades. Depression. Doing little things such as the laundry feels like an uphill battle. My jerky movements come from spurts of energy squeezed from my nearly lifeless hulk. I am devolving into myself, weary, purposeless, submerged in a world filled with muffled echoes of my own thoughts and the whispers of others, a dark and desolate world. As my mind congeals, my speech slows. I petrify.

A simple sign that I am depressed is that I won't answer the phone. With a few loud epithets, I threw it from my bedroom window one evening. To me, the action was justified. Each time the phone rang, my hypersensitive hearing magnified the sound. Edgar Allan Poe's protagonist in "The Tell-Tale Heart" could have been speaking for me when he protested, "And have I not told you that what you mistake for madness is but overacuteness of the senses?" In this state, I see phone calls either as an attack or a trick to control my time. As an act of self-protection, I refuse to let them in. By contrast, a simple sign that I am "cycling" back into a manic mood is that you can't get me off the phone. I use the term *cycling* to mean transitioning from one mood or energy state into another—for example, a bounce from a nonenergized state into a mania or a crash from mania into depression.

When manic, I can't tell the difference between the world changing around me and my perception of it changing from within, and the boundaries between me and the world begin to blur. As my mind escalates into mania, I whirl into extended moments of free association, as in the poem at the beginning of this chapter. The link between ideas extends beyond their substance to their sounds. Words assume color and rush to fuse with those of like hue. This is a world of heightened sensitivity to movement, to shape, to sound. It is a sleepless time, exploding with previously untapped energies. Tireless days give way to energy-filled nights. Ask me how I think others see me and I will tell you they see me as brilliant, creative, alliterative, witty, and as mentally acute as I'm capable of being. It is an exhilarating time.

What does depression feel like? I become a 120-year-old man. I have no energy; I slump when I sit and take small steps when

I move. When I eat, I eat little and chew slowly. I am conscious of the sound of my breathing.

Walking someplace is difficult. As a coping technique, I shadow someone in front of me and let them tow me along. Step after step, inch after inch, I walk in straight lines using all my energy to follow the pavement's edge. Those passing by seem to be deliberately jostling me, bumping shoulders, encroaching on my space.

When experiencing a manic or depressive episode, I assign negative meaning to innocent cues; strangers seem menacing. I conclude that the cashier at 7-Eleven means the opposite when she says, "Have a nice day," and hands me my change for a bottle of juice. My attention is drawn to things that are disturbing, like a homeless person on the street or a badly dented car. When truck drivers blast their horns, I think they are doing it to aggravate me.

When depressed I do my best to hide it. Ask me how I am feeling and I'll respond that I am just tired. Sometimes it's true and that's all there is to it. But something *When depressed I do my best to hide it.* more is going on, like when I avoid eye contact and slur my speech, sleep for much longer than usual, refuse to initiate conversations, and retreat into isolation.

When I'm depressed, my head feels thick. I've gotten this feeling with each episode. When it occurs, I know I should have gotten help sooner. Now, after years of monitoring, I recognize it as a sign of my descent into depression. I now recognize many signs that warn of the onset of either mood/energy state. Where mania is previewed by an increasing sense of power, depression is forecasted by an escalating sense of powerlessness. Where mania is bright, depression is dull. Mania is a process of acceleration, depression of deceleration. Regular visits with a mental health professional seemed like torture when I was a teen and had other priorities, but they helped ward off the uglier manifestations of the illness because I learned more about what my warning signs were and what action to take to get help.

When I'm in a mania, I take unnecessary risks and am not accommodating to others. When I was old enough to know better but my mood and energy were cycling unchecked, a black sport utility vehicle revved its engine and squealed its tires before tearing past me on a road that had no sidewalk. Thinking it had tried to run me over, I threw a paper cup with the remains of a soda at the menacing vehicle and hit my target. Now I know that it is really stupid to throw things at moving vehicles—especially an ill-tempered martial artist's truck. Violent beginnings have violent ends. The driver chased me on foot and punched me in the throat. Another time, I destroyed a VCR while thinking that if I could change its shape, it would fit in my suitcase for an upcoming trip. I don't remember what I thought that would accomplish, but at the time it all made perfect sense to me. Parents don't take kindly to home electronics destruction.

During one manic episode, I followed the turn signals of the car ahead of me for direction because I thought God was trying to lead me. But mania sparks second and third interpretations for every action. Alternatively, I thought following the car ahead of me would reveal something important and otherwise unknowable, a mystery unraveled—where that car was going.

Once, when manic at my Quaker high school's meeting for worship, I couldn't sit quietly any longer, so I stood up and blurted out that the school's refusal to display certain works of art was no different from Nazi censorship of the opponents of fascism. I succeeded in practicing public speaking and in aggravating a lot of teachers. It's easy to make a fool of yourself when classmates and teachers hear you free associate at lightning speed. It may win poetry contests, but it looks and sounds weird.

A Literary-Minded Delusion

At times when I was mood and energy cycling I experienced another possible symptom of bipolar disorder, what psychiatrists call *psychotic features*, including a delusion that inflated my sense of self worth. In the world of mental health, people are considered psychotic who have trouble dealing with their environment in part because of delusions (false beliefs) and hallucinations (false sensory perceptions). For example, at times I've felt as though I've been attacked. Sometimes others' realities defined mine. Once I was trapped in George Orwell's novel *1984*. The government was Big Brother, and police officers and teachers were agents of the state, monitoring me. It is hard to break from this way of thinking because *1984* is plausible. The state does spy on its own people. What helped me escape my Orwellian trap was the realization that the state doesn't focus on 16-year-old high school kids unless they are murderers, championship gymnasts, or really good hackers. I was none of the above. Why would someone spend money to have me watched, part of my mind asked? But then again, another part of my mind argued, what if Big Brother had planted that question?

Sometimes when manic I feel as if I am from another time. In one mania I lived in the Philadelphia of the future at the same time that my body walked down the streets of the Philadelphia

> . . . people are considered psychotic who have trouble dealing with their environment in part because of delusions and hallucinations . . .

of the present. Everything seemed 20 years from now. I didn't realize it at the time, but it is not safe for me to be alone when my sense of reality is so distorted. Usually when my world accelerates, I just ride it out. But it was difficult this time. I was, after all, in the future without familiar landmarks. When I approached strangers for help, they hurried away with fear in their eyes. I couldn't find my green Volkswagen Rabbit. I wandered wet, black paved streets. Steam from metal sewer vents transformed a neon sign's red letters into hieroglyphs, and the sounds of sirens and car tires, passersby and pigeons, fused into one symphony. A page of newspaper blew across the boulevard and up a stone wall only to float back down for another ride. If there was a God in this world, I wanted to be remembered, so I dropped a quarter in a homeless man's cup. I passed a bolted church. If God was not already inside, he would have trouble getting in, I thought.

Instinct carried me from the middle of Center City Philadelphia back to my home just inside the edge of the city (drop me anywhere within walking distance of a transit stop and I can sleepwalk my way through the transit system). When I arrived home, my parents were awake. My friend Hector had called them when I failed to arrive at his apartment. He had organized a group that went out searching for me. I assured my parents I was okay: I just couldn't remember where Hector lived or where I had parked the car, and so I took the train home. The following morning I called my psychiatrist for an emergency meeting at which he adjusted my medication. My mind calmed, and I returned to living in the present.

A Quick Reflection

When I'm manic there is always more than one possible explanation for everything and anything. Perhaps this has something to do with the inspiration artists associate with their highly creative periods. Some experiences don't translate well into words. As strange as it sounds, in a manic state truths are paradoxes, yet for once the universe makes total sense. You've got creative energy to burn. Things don't become uncomfortable until your pleasure-filled mania splinters into a psychotic mess.

When I'm psychotic, I am irritable and have little tolerance of others. Getting bumped on the sidewalk or cut off by another driver can escalate into a shouting match or worse. The times in my life when I have been closest to going to jail have happened during psychotic episodes. The good news is that I had health insurance and was able to recover from psychotic breaks in psychiatric wards.

If you have experienced mania or depression, you know what the words mean. If you haven't, the best you can do is empathize. Once you have felt psychotically manic or clinically depressed, you don't want to go through it again. And if medication and the mentoring of doctors, families, and friends don't head off a second or third experience, you want the next time to be shorter and the journey less difficult. The good news is that there may not be a next time and, if there is, you have ways of coping that you lacked the first time it hit. You now know your enemy's name and know as well that it can be tamed by medication, psychotherapy, and the support of those who love you and whom you love.

> If you have experienced mania or depression, you know what the words mean. If you haven't, the best you can do is empathize.

Chapter Two

How It All Began

It is as if my life were magically run by two electric currents: joyous positive and despairing negative—whichever is running at the moment dominates my life, floods it.

> —Sylvia Plath, who had manic-depressive illness,
> *The Unabridged Journals of Sylvia Plath* (2000)

Oahu, Hawaii

I experienced my first manic episode at 11, just after my family moved from Maryland to Hawaii for six months. I found Hawaii dizzyingly bright, a world of billowing white clouds and blue ocean. It was there that I felt for the first time a heightened sense of energy, a reduced need for sleep, and an accelerated rush of thought and speech. No one thought anything of it. To my parents, these behaviors looked like a reasonable response to a new place filled with sun and surf. But something wasn't right, because I felt on edge and angry.

The year-round flowers and flowering plants also triggered my asthma and I started wheezing. I was taken to an asthma specialist, who sent me home with a cortisone-based inhalant—which at the time was new but now is standard treatment. Within half a day of the first breath of the inhalant, the world crashed around me. Feeling worthless, hopeless, frightened, and alone, I recoiled from those around me. Watching my retreat with alarm, my mother discontinued the inhalant and called the doctor to report that it had produced a bizarre effect. She said, "In an adult I would call Patrick's response depression." In fact, after three months of mania probably activated by the stress of the move, I was now experiencing, as an 11-year-old, a full-blown drug crash that looked just like depression—seemingly brought on by a rare reaction to the cortisone in the inhalant. Years later, a doctor told me it was probably a coincidence, but in any event it didn't last long and my mood leveled off for the rest of the time in Hawaii. Nonetheless, I remember my stay there as a disturbing and troubled time—paradise lost.

Austin, Texas

When I was 13 years old, after a brief interlude back in Maryland, my family moved again, this time to Austin, Texas. Several months later, I started having health problems. My allergies were acting up. I picked up several sinus infections, then bronchitis. I was tired but mistakenly shrugged off my lethargy as a consequence of the bronchitis. The thought that I might be depressed never crossed the minds of my parents or any of the doctors they sought out. My reputation as an eccentric, based in the free-wheeling individualism cultivated by a Montessori education and an anti-authoritarian upbringing reinforced by my parents, explained any symptoms of mental illness. Just like my mother, who had assumed that whatever the cortisone-based inhalant was doing to me, it could not have been triggering depression in an 11-year-old. I had no idea teenagers were susceptible to depression at all, much less manic depression. Indeed, at that point, I don't think I'd ever heard manic and depression combined into a single term.

I had no idea teenagers were susceptible to depression at all, much less manic depression.

In Austin I felt like a stranger in a strange land. Texas: big refrigerators, BBQ smokehouses, and dry 104-degree Augusts. During the school year, weekends slip by too fast and Monday mornings come much too soon. My experience was this: I don't sleep well. My cat's fleas find me an appealing alternative and the air conditioner's cycle disturbs my sleep. I wake up groggy. My chest feels hollow. My heart pounds. I've slept through my alarm clock again and am late for school.

In the car en route to school, I realize that something primitive has taken hold of me. My thoughts are spinning. My brain has shifted from first to fourth gear. At school, I stare transfixed in front of my locker as a crush of students shuffles around me to classes. My left hand is gripping my protractor, tangible evidence that I am enrolled in a geometry class, but I do not remember removing it from my backpack. My thoughts have moved from a trot to a full, all-out gallop and from the concrete world around me to fanciful abstraction. If my life is ordinarily a photograph, today it is like a Van Gogh with intense color and distorted perspective.

English class is a blur. I can't focus well enough to take notes. I write silliness. "Hour Father. Lettuce prey." I obscure page after page with intersecting lines. I recall the stitching on one of my aunt's pillows, "God writes straight with crooked lines." There's nothing straight about today.

In geometry class, the representations on the board morph into artistic shapes. The two-dimensional has assumed a third dimension. The rectangle on the board is a toy box, a coffin, the transport vehicle of the starship *Enterprise*. I answer the teacher's questions absurdly. The area under the curve, I proclaim, is the negative space revealed by drawing a rectangle around the formula. The teacher has long ago written me off as a smart-ass. I create similar scenarios in later classes.

During the bus ride home, a classmate repeatedly pokes fun at my uncombed hair. "You're a slob," the ferret-faced preppy with wire-rim glasses says, his beady blue eyes in razor focus. Ordinarily I'd retaliate with a clever put-down, but my mind won't muster one. It is speeding on to something else. I mutter what those of delicate sensibilities would call an expletive. I relive this fragmented exchange late into the night. Instead of an incidental conversation, it becomes a full-blown morality play, or a confrontation between Wile E. Coyote and the Roadrunner—except in this scenario, the Roadrunner is uncharacteristically dragging a heavy ball and chain.

Trying to slow my thoughts tightens the leash around my neck. Have you ever tried to force yourself to be calm in bed at night when something catastrophic has happened? A relative has died. You've been in a car accident. It's impossible. My thoughts penetrate every barrier constructed to contain them. I once thought that with practice I could learn to control my thoughts when manic. That was an illusion.

In my experience, manias often forecast depression. The danger and deadliness of each are magnified when they combine to form what psychiatrists call a *mixed state*—a time when both manic and depressed symptoms surface. Years later I would recognize that my experience in Austin—the fast thoughts, lack of focus, and low energy—was a mixed state. For me, it is the most uncomfortable state to be in because it makes relating to others more difficult. My thinking is unhinged from the here and now. It's a lose-lose situation for everybody. But at the time, I had no idea what was going on. Maybe this is what it felt like to be a teenager, I thought. Maybe all of this is hormonal.

Maybe this is what it felt like to be a teenager, I thought. Maybe all of this is hormonal.

Others around me were bewildered as well. During this extended period of mania followed by depression and a mixed state, my parents and I met with doctor after doctor in Austin. I was poked and probed, scanned and scrutinized. It seemed as if every bodily fluid of mine that could be extracted was tested for diseases both rare and common. After battery upon battery of tests, each doctor offered a different diagnosis. An immune system disorder, reported one. A rare form of mononucleosis, concluded another. Epstein-Barr syndrome, said a third. Allergies, proclaimed a fourth. None could produce a blood or urine test, a CT scan or MRI showing any tangible evidence for these diagnoses. They might as well have said, "We haven't got a clue."

Exhausted after months of little sleep and still less focus, I crashed out of the mixed state and into a five-month depression during which I slept up to 18 hours a day and missed more school than I attended. I started feeling well just in time to study enough to squeak past finals. As that process drew to a close, I spent increasing amounts of time with a mallet in hand, working on the timber-frame addition to our family house that my father was building outside my bedroom window.

The satisfaction of building something by hand was primitive. I sharpened my own chisels and made my own mallets. It felt good to step back and survey what I had accomplished at the end of the day, the week, and the month. Part of me was in the house. The process also felt therapeutic. The strength in my hands, arms, and shoulders seemed to carry over to my brain. Driving pegs into the wooden joints to lock them in place focused my mind.

A friend of my dad's named Jon helped with the heavy work. What I knew about him was limited to the scattered fragments of information that slipped out in conversations among adults. If he took his medication, said the whispers of adults, he was fine. When he felt well, however, he'd occasionally stop the medication and ultimately required hospitalization. His illness was called bipolar disorder.

Considered brilliant in college, he had not held a steady job since. After some sort of "breakdown," he was given lithium, a mood-stabilizing medication. I feared him at first because I didn't know what to expect from someone who had to take lithium. Around me, he seemed as normal as any other adult, married with two kids, quick, witty, and unaffected by the ultimate adult sin: He was not patronizing. At first the mystery surrounding his illness frightened me. Working on the roof of the three-story timber frame put us more than 27 feet above the ground. How safe was it to be up there with someone with a mental disorder, I wondered. The doubts evaporated quickly. He worked as hard as my dad did. They were friends. He was a good guy. What I did not know at the time was that he and his wife had seen a parallel between my highs and lows of the past academic year and Jon's own journey into bipolar disorder.

Contact with Jon was not my only early encounter with bipolar disorder. My aunt's husband, Kyle, was a charismatic, all-around guy who loved gourmet cooking, camping in the woods, whitewater rafting, canoeing, and roughing it in the wild. He also wrote music and played saxophone and rhythm guitar in a rock band. To me, he became living proof that the boring adult lives forecast by our parents—as engineers, lawyers, doctors, or professors—were not the inevitable end of growing up.

But there was another Kyle. The first hint of this side of him came when he failed to attend a family reunion at my grandparents'. Rumors circulated through the family. Kyle had spent months in silence in a darkened room. He had not returned home for days while engaged in marathon recording sessions with his band. This Kyle used uppers to counter his depression and downers to dampen his mania, a common practice for people with bipolar disorder. This Kyle refused my aunt's pleas to see a doctor and take prescribed medication for bipolar disorder. Faced with an ultimatum, therapy and medication or divorce, Kyle chose divorce. After that his drinking and drug use escalated. Years later, unable to lift himself from a deep depression, and unwilling to seek help, he killed himself.

I remember Kyle during a canoeing trip, when he vaulted from his canoe to help my brother and me right ours after it capsized. I remember Kyle's ludicrous story about a headless ghoul and his joking about it as he helped us build the campfire that would cook our dinner. I did not know the Kyle who ended his own life. Or perhaps I did but didn't understand.

Philadelphia, Pennsylvania

We left Austin in 1989, this time moving to Philadelphia, where I was enrolled as a sophomore in a private urban Quaker school. I was 15, and by late summer I had been transformed from someone who slept more than most to someone who didn't seem to need to sleep at all. My energy was back. That fall I had a full course load—history, English, French, and my worst subject, algebra 2—and I fell behind almost from the start. My mind was racing and my ability to focus in class came and went. The school principal called my mother. "We are concerned about Patrick," she said. "He isn't focusing, his speech is rapid, he's not making a lot of sense. I think you should take him to a doctor."

After three years in Austin, the move to Philadelphia had put me and my family in touch with a local medical teaching hospital, and with it experts who not only recognized but also studied adolescent bipolar disorder. Confronted with a 15-year-old who hadn't slept in days, could not control his thoughts, and was increasingly verbally aggressive, my primary care physician at the hospital offered two hypotheses—a thyroid malfunction or bipolar disorder. The doctors in Austin had already checked for a thyroid malfunction and found none. A blood test confirmed their conclusion, leaving a diagnosis of bipolar disorder.

When I asked if that meant that I was schizophrenic, the only label of mental illness I could readily summon, the doctor clearly ruled it out. Now I know that it is sometimes difficult to draw a line between mood or "affective" disorders like bipolar disorder and schizophrenia. Indeed, there are cases in which individuals have the symptoms of both and are diagnosed as schizoaffective.

Later, my middle-aged parents sat with me in the Youth Guidance Center, next to a middle-aged male psychiatrist with short black hair, glasses, and a graying beard. Dr. Gottstein said, "There's a good chance we're dealing with manic depression or bipolar disorder." My reaction is the same as it was when the diagnosis was first offered by my family doctor. I am stunned. Five minutes later my disbelief is still bristling. He can't be right, I think, there's nothing wrong with me but Epstein-Barr syndrome or an immune disorder. That was what the doctors in Austin had said, and I now desperately wanted to believe them. My symptoms are real. They are physical. My heart is racing. My throat is dry. This is not all in my head, I repeat to myself. I am not "mental." I am not crazy.

> My reaction is the same as it was when the diagnosis was first offered by my family doctor. I am stunned.

If I was ill, I wanted a physical illness, not a mental illness—and I resolutely believed at the time that there was a clean distinction between the two. I wanted an illness caused by a bacterium that could be treated with an antibiotic or one produced by a splinter that could be removed by surgery. Psychiatric illness wasn't real; it was "all in your head"—the ultimate form of self-indulgent hypochondria, I thought, a copout for those too lazy or inept to cope with the world, a con used to bilk insurance companies and trick employers.

If it is difficult at 15 to accept a chronic illness, it is even more difficult to accept one about which much is unknown. When bipolar disorder entered my vocabulary, years after it had entered my life, I believed the stereotypes of so-called "mental illness" as much as anyone else. And one of the insidious things about stereotypes is that you think they are facts. I started trying to find information that would make sense to me and would reveal what about this condition was fact and what was fantasy. I wanted to know what this diagnosis meant for me. But the problem is that, although researchers and doctors have made great strides in understanding and treating bipolar disorder, there is still much that remains unknown about the illness, especially in adolescents, an understudied population. And so, some of what I found answered my questions, while other materials raised more concerns than they quieted.

As it was, the doctor addressing my family was a psychiatrist specializing in treatment of adolescents with bipolar disorder. I didn't want him to be right. I didn't want the stigma of a "mental illness." And I didn't want the treatment. "If this is bipolar disorder, you'll have to take lithium for the rest of your life," he said. I thought, "It's impossible! I can't even brush my teeth twice a day." I picked up fragments of what he was saying. No beer. No booze. No drugs. No dope. Weekly appointments. I felt 15 going on 40. From now on I was supposed to act grown up. I felt cheated out of being a teenager.

Although they are slowly changing, widespread Western societal stereotypes hold that being physically ill is preferable to being mentally ill, seeing a minister is better than seeing a psychotherapist, seeing a psychotherapist is better than seeing a psychiatrist, being treated as an outpatient is preferable to being treated as an inpatient, and voluntary hospitalization is preferred to involuntary hospitalization. Unfortunately, many of us deny our own conditions, even to ourselves.

Seeing a psychiatrist seemed to be an admission that I was crazy. I resented his presuming to interpret my attitudes and behavior. I resented the assumption that I was abusing alcohol and street drugs. My resentment took the form of sarcastic and sometimes savage words and a war of wills. I responded to a difficult situation by blaming my predicament on my "shrink" (as I referred to him when I was angry).

My belief that I didn't need anybody's help added to my disdain for psychiatrists. Asking for help seemed to me a sign of weakness. I was also hard on myself for not being able to solve my own problems. I felt incompetent for having to rely on a doctor and a hospital bed as tools for staying alive. Maybe this self-reliance is a macho male weakness. Like the great baseball star Joe DiMaggio, men are supposed to be able to play with pain. This thinking got me into trouble when I felt fine for an extended period, decided I had either been misdiagnosed or cured, stopped taking lithium, and relapsed.

Another reason that I disliked psychiatrists was that I associated them with the seemingly endless urine samples and blood tests a freshly diagnosed person encounters when attempting to get new medications balanced. I couldn't walk out of my doc's office without new prescriptions in hand. I also associated him with long lines and large bills. (Insurance that covers 100% of a so-called physical illness will often cover only half of the cost of a so-called mental one.)

As much as I resented having bipolar disorder, and having to take medication for it, I resisted even more the "talk" sessions of psychotherapy. Teenagers take privacy very seriously. These are years in which our bedrooms are off limits even to family members, years in which phone conversations with friends take on a conspiratorial tone. Into this walled-off world comes a prying adult asking very personal questions: questions about feelings and family, questions about drugs and alcohol, questions about sexual inclinations and actions, questions about sleep patterns and thoughts of suicide. The questions are troubling in part because they suggest the range of concerns that have come to preoccupy those around you.

Every query by the psychiatrist who diagnosed my condition (I had not yet awarded him the status of "my" psychiatrist) seemed like prying. I've known those who will tell anyone anything; I've never been one of them. I make friends cautiously and share confidences hesitantly. Although his attitude was nonjudgmental, the psychiatrist's questions seemed to me to be invasive. He had not earned the right to ask. I didn't trust him enough to answer.

. . . the psychiatrist's questions seemed to me to be invasive. He had not earned the right to ask. I didn't trust him enough to answer.

I also didn't like having to be self-reflective on command and rebelled against the requirements of the so-called "medication management" sessions. I needed someone to blame for my anger, fear, and disbelief. True to the profile sketched by the psychology manuals, I blamed my doc.

Psychiatrists are trained to ask questions rather than to give answers. Psychiatry blends science and art to address an individual with a unique personal history. It is one of the most difficult professions around. Psychiatrists are medical school graduates with extensive residency experience. Like trauma surgeons, they keep people alive, but unlike trauma surgeons, they see their patients for weeks, months, or years. While some doctors can think of a patient as an occasional office visitor, a psychiatrist has an ongoing therapeutic relationship with a client, with the client relying on that relationship for guidance in life survival skills.

Adolescents inherit more than an illness when they are diagnosed with bipolar disorder. We have to deal with frightened parents and, once diagnosed, we have to navigate a relationship with even more adults, including a psychiatrist or therapist. Teen bipolar disorder is a family problem that affects siblings and spouses, as well as parents and grandparents. To the extent that they will be called on to help us manage this disorder, they need to be brought into a relationship with the managing doctor as well.

At 16 I had a more cynical view of the client-psychiatrist relationship than I do now. I didn't think psychiatrists deserved the insurance money they were claiming for "doing nothing." I didn't think it was fair to pay my psychiatrist well over $100 every two weeks or every month to secure a prescription. Why couldn't he just phone in the prescription or give me a standing order?

Now I know that my relapse rate is much lower because I see a psychiatrist regularly. The National Institute of Mental Health says, "Studies have shown that psychosocial interventions can lead to increased mood stability, fewer hospitalizations, and improved functioning in several areas." In other words, seeing a therapist or psychiatrist is important.

Bipolar 101

With lithium comes lithium monitoring. Life became framed by the white walls of the outpatient clinic and the hospital that

I visited on a regular basis. After a few months I could navigate the outpatient section of my mental health facility blindfolded. I took blood tests every two weeks to permit my doctor to monitor my lithium level and gave urine samples for reasons that were not clear to me. I'm lucky that I've got thick veins close to the surface. I switched arms each time and kidded as my blood was drawn. Realizing that humor masks fear, the phlebotomists smiled as if they were hearing the questions for the first time, "Do you think I'll run out?" "Is it still red?" But there is nothing funny about the process. More than once, bad technique and a misplaced needle left me blood-bruised from elbow to wrist. It looks scary but isn't dangerous. Bad blood-drawing technique is just one fact of life with any chronic illness.

I became a pro at providing urine samples. I envisioned competing in the pee-in-the-cup relay at the next bipolar Olympic Games. For males, the technique is all in the wrist. Here we go again! I rolled up my sleeve, ran the cold water on my wrist, threw away the towelette wrapper, unzipped, pissed, let the cup hold the stream for a second, finished peeing, zipped up, found the receiving tray, and headed out to pay the bill. An alternative competition would be hurling into the trash those little antiseptic towelette packets dispensed with each urine container. And when the world goes awry, there's always the pole vault over the asylum wall. (Those of us with a so-called "mental illness" can joke about the asylum; those who love us should do so with great hesitation.)

At the time, no one told me that in addition to checking my lithium level, someone in a white smock somewhere was checking for illegal drugs, including THC, a product stored in the fat of marijuana users. Because those with bipolar disorder are likely to abuse alcohol and street drugs, and because either can undercut treatment, the doctors, in the words of a

Because those with bipolar disorder are likely to abuse alcohol and street drugs, and because either can undercut treatment, the doctors, in the words of a former U.S. president, "trust but verify."

former U.S. president, "trust but verify." Since I wasn't doing drugs or drinking at the time of diagnosis, I resented the assumption that verification was needed. Why not take me at my word?

So: Not only did I have to take lithium every day—pills in the morning and pills at night—as if I were in a nursing home, I had to learn to live both with the fact that I wouldn't be able to drink at any age and with the assumption by doctors that I would self-medicate with pot and alcohol anyway. I wanted credit for making a good-faith effort to cope with this illness, and no credit was given. Now I realize that instead of being insulted, I should have felt complimented that my psychiatrist assumed I was smart enough to hide any consumption of alcohol or drug abuse from even conscientious parents and a vigilant shrink. Later I would prove to my parents, my doctors, and myself that I was indeed clever enough to camouflage drinking. What I could conceal from them I couldn't hide from my brain, however, which rewarded my behavior with a "lithium breakthrough" and a hospitalization. In science, a breakthrough is an accomplishment; when tied to lithium, though, the metaphor is a synonym for failure: The illness had "broken through" the lithium.

Being a teenager is hard enough without having to negotiate a chronic medical condition. You've just learned to drive, but your disorientation is causing doubts about whether you should. The older guys are dating all the girls your age, especially the pretty ones with brains, leaving few for you. Your grades are bad, so bad you might have to go to summer school, the only thing worse than a minimum-wage summer job mowing lawns.

But after being diagnosed with bipolar disorder my first semester in Philadelphia and going on lithium, I stabilized. The wild energy swings had been tamed. Maybe I was going to be all right, I thought. Soon, spring arrived. A friend back in Austin, Beth, was fighting to graduate first in her class at Austin High School. A so-so student, I was impressed. I wrote her every week. We occasionally spoke by phone. One night, she called to ask, "Patrick, will you fly down to Texas and be my prom date in April?" I responded, "Are you serious? YOU BET I WILL!" I knew that we were just friends. But even friends can hope.

By spring it was clear that I was only a partial responder to lithium. It worked, but not well enough to completely control the highs and lows. By early April I had entered another mixed state—my mind was on fast-forward and my body was on rewind. Adjustments in medication didn't break the mixed state. I was disoriented. My parents recommended that I call Beth to explain that I was too ill to fly to Austin for the prom. I couldn't bring myself to do it. Someone important to me was counting on me. There had to be a way. With my ticket in one hand and suitcase in the other, I went to catch the train to the airport. Thanks to a drug-induced sleep the past night, I felt detached from reality, but halfway to the train station, I realized that I wasn't sufficiently in control to dance and because of the lithium could not drink at the prom. I trudged back home, dropped my suitcase, slogged up the stairs to my bedroom, curled up in a ball on my messy bed, and wished that I could hurl this damned disorder into outer space.

Once you are diagnosed with bipolar disorder, it feels as if life is conspiring against you. Your parents and shrink watch you like hawks eyeing a pigeon. You aren't given any space. Your teachers say you've got enormous potential while dumping

C's onto your transcript. A lot of your problem is that you've been functioning with a chronic condition without knowing or treating it. Now everyone in your life has to figure out what this condition means. Not knowing how means that a lot of people are overreacting. Or so it seems to you.

People with bipolar disorder can have long periods of remission. During one such period of normal functioning, I had many of the same experiences of adolescence as others my age. By my logic at the time, I either had been cured or hadn't actually had bipolar disorder to begin with. So, with new friends I made on the soccer and baseball teams, I partied throughout the summer before the best year of my high school career, junior year, while restricting my intake of alcohol. Unfortunately, this period of "normalcy" was short-lived and led me into a false sense of confidence. Feeling super-charged and sensing no difference between my responses to the world and those of my friends, I then did what half of all lithium users do and stopped taking the medication. I did not talk to my parents about my rash decision to quit the medication because I knew they would try to stop me. Had I known that for a significant percentage of those who quit the medication, lithium won't work in the future, I might have made a different decision.

Because I was off lithium I no longer needed to worry about the effect of alcohol on my lithium level. Presumably now I could drink beer with no ill effects. As someone on the cusp of 17, drinking with the guys was a rite of passage I wanted to share. Then in October the gods created the sort of opportunity for which an adolescent prays. Looking innocent and sounding responsible, I persuaded my parents that I should be left at home to take care of the pets—two cats and a dog—while they attended a meeting in Atlanta. I was after all 17, one year away from voting and registering for the draft. The con worked.

Marshaling the skill and energies of two of my friends and squandering the money I had earned over the summer, I staged a blow-out party worthy of the movie *Animal House*: Multiple kegs, multiple cases of beer, cartons of Pepsi, party favors, cigars, balloons, party food, and 30 of my closest friends. Those with connections brought other ingredients.

The bash began at 7 P.M. on a Saturday evening. The first hour was quiet. Some stood around and talked. Others danced in the living room. A couple necked on the couch. Some were drinking beer, others soda. My preference was beer. As the blood alcohol levels of my guests rose, my control over the party dropped. At around 9, the tone began to change. When three juniors rammed Slayer and Metallica discs into my CD player, the decibel level jumped. The girls who had been dancing in our living room responded by fleeing to other rooms.

A friend asked me to start our 15-year-old orange riding lawn mower, and being too drunk to distinguish a good idea from a bad one, I did. I had become a drunken fifth horseman of the apocalypse. Death, war, famine, pestilence, and inebriation. After careening around the yard, headlights shattering the darkness, I crashed through the wooden trellises surrounding our porches and ended my driving for the night.

Inside, a 240-pound friend had demonstrated his talent as a Jackie Chan wannabe by smashing his arm and fist through our kitchen table. Splinters fell to the floor as if it were a movie prop.

As party meister, I had filled one super soaker squirt gun with vodka and the other with tonic water. By 10 P.M., the guns were empty. Meanwhile, the party had grown from the 30 we had invited to 150, many of them party crashers from a neighboring school. The music, the clash of voices, and the crush of people increased dramatically.

Concerned about the noise and recognizing that the house was in shambles, I shut the party down at 2:30 A.M., by announcing that a neighbor had called the police. Three classmates who were clearly too drunk to drive home crashed on couches and the floor for the night. Another classmate drove me to a 24-hour Dunkin' Donuts for my first nonalcoholic meal since noon: chicken noodle soup and a glazed donut. Upon our return, I checked again on those sleeping on the floor and started the process of cleaning up. It was at that point that I noticed that the front and back doors of the house were propped open. The dog and two cats were gone. The next day I would learn that my mother's jewelry was gone as well.

My parents returned Sunday around noon to a hollowed-out distillery they had once called home and a handful of my hungover friends valiantly trying to erase evidence of the night's partying. I had hidden eight disposable lawn and leaf sacks full of party garbage behind the wood pile but hadn't had time to air out the house completely or scour the eighth of an inch of crud off the oak living room floor. Although two friends and I had mopped the floors, the house reeked of vomit.

The price I paid for this major infraction was small. I was grounded for six months and had to clean everything and replace anything that had been broken. And fortunately, the dog, cats, and jewelry were all eventually retrieved. In hindsight I see the party was a really bad idea, but had I been medicated, I might have hosted it anyway. The peer pressure I faced was strong, and I very much wanted to remain popular with my new friends at school who had hosted similar parties. Mostly I wanted to feel like every other kid my age and being a party animal seemed a good way to accomplish that goal.

As fall became winter and the slush-saturated leaves made the edges of the streets slick, my energy subsided and I fell into a depression. As I slowed so did my sense of the passage of time. Unfinished homework piled up on my desk. Seeing a hospitalization in my future if I didn't correct course quickly, in consultation with my doctor I went back on lithium. Since lithium is better at preventing the ups than it is the downs in cycles, it took weeks to feel better. Slowly I felt equilibrium return.

But as months passed it became clearer that lithium alone wasn't completely keeping my bipolar disorder at bay. My psychiatrist suggested adding another drug and asked me to pick one of two new anticonvulsant medications that could help stabilize my mood. Having received no clear evidence from him which was better, I made my choice. After several days on my new med, my skin turned pink and red as if I was scalded in a steaming hot shower, and it started sloughing off. I threw up repeatedly each time I tried to eat. I convinced my parents that people with the flu don't turn red and lose their skin, and we sought medical attention.

> . . . it became clearer that lithium alone wasn't completely keeping my bipolar disorder at bay.

I was diagnosed as having a Stevens-Johnson type affliction, an extremely rare allergic reaction caused by the new medication. After taking steroids that I was warned would make me manic (better than being dead, I thought) and an unwelcome 32-day excursion to the hospital, I went home. I was told that I had to quit drinking alcohol because my liver was scarred from the allergic reaction. In other words, if you start a new medication, watch for allergic reactions and chemical interactions that your prescriber may not warn you about or even expect.

The Catcher in the Rye's Holden Caulfield and Manic Depression

Medicated or not, some of my high school experiences were dissimilar from those of my peers. When I read J. D. Salinger's novel *The Catcher in the Rye* (1951) during my junior year, parts seemed eerily familiar. Holden's bipolar, I thought. How else to explain the fact that he is hostile, listless, lethargic, disinterested, and, before Darth Vader altered the meaning of the phrase, focused on the dark side. For Holden, the traumatic event that may have kindled the illness was the death of his younger brother, Allie. He reacts by breaking windows with his bare hands and is hospitalized as a result. Although the text is not explicit, that hospital may have been a psychiatric institution. The illness he experiences on his return home is psychological.

He is also suicidal, spends a lot of time on the phone, places calls late at night, has trouble sleeping, speaks too loudly, cries without motivation, reports repeatedly that he is depressed, and spends money indiscriminately. Additionally, he is a heavy smoker, which may be his means of self-medication. Also, he experiences a disconnection between feeling and action. "I felt like praying or something, when I was in bed, but I couldn't do it. I can't always pray when I feel like it." Finally, he has contradictory feelings at the same time. "I didn't even like her much and yet all of a sudden I felt I was in love with her and wanted to marry her," he says of the character Sally.

Holden's rapid speech and disconnected conversations are signs of mania. When conversing with Sally, he says, "Take most people, they're crazy about cars. They worry if they get a little scratch on them, and they're always talking about how many miles they get to a gallon, and if they get a brand-new car already they start thinking about trading it in for one that's even newer. I don't even like old cars. I mean they don't even interest me. I'd rather have goddam horse. A horse is at least human." Sally responds, "I don't know what you're even talking about. . . . You just jump from one—."

If Holden were suffering from bipolar disorder in the 1950s, when the book appeared, his future was less optimistic than it would be were he diagnosed today. Lithium, which stabilizes the chemical imbalance that causes bipolar disorder, was not approved for use in the United States until 1970. Without lithium, Holden would likely continue to experience mood swings and possibly take his own life. Those with severe psychiatric disorders are roughly seven to ten times more likely to kill themselves than is the general population. But treatment works, and one study done in 2002 reported that treated patients had less than half the suicide rate of those who had not been treated. Fortunately for Holden, many with the illness also experience extended periods free of symptoms. I have.

In the 1950s, when *Catcher* appeared, most psychiatrists would not have made the diagnosis of bipolar disorder. In fact, under the spell of Sigmund Freud and his heirs, Holden wouldn't have even been labeled mentally ill. According to the orthodoxy of the time, teens weren't developmentally advanced enough to be able to internalize anger or experience depression. Freud divided the mind into three categories: ego, superego, and id. For Freudians, since a punishing superego prompted depression, and kids didn't yet have a superego, kids couldn't be depressed. As you may know from sophomore English, that's the same Freud who fathered the Oedipus complex (whether he fathered it by sleeping with his mother is another question). If Oedipus became desolate and sleepless in Athens because he realized that wanting to kill his father and sleep with his mother was a genuinely nutty idea, then according to Freud, he would have had to wait for the development of his superego to earn the label "depressed." Thankfully, this theory has been debunked and doctors know a lot more about adolescence and mood disorders in young people, and they have better treatments now than they did in the 1950s. The next chapter is a brief look at what they know.

Chapter Three

What Do Doctors Know About Bipolar Disorder and How Do They Know It?

The war that I waged against myself is not an uncommon one. The major clinical problem in treating manic depression is not that there are not effective medications, because there are, but that patients so often refuse to take them. Worse yet, because of a lack of information, poor medical advice, poor medical treatment, terrible stigma or fear of personal and professional reprisals, patients do not seek treatment at all.

—Dr. Kay Redfield Jamison, "Manic Depression:
A Personal and Professional Perspective," speech given on
July 26, 2000, at the University of Melbourne in Australia

How are you today?" the doctor asks. Your throat is sore. Swallowing feels like trying to down a prickly pear. You're running a fever. "I think I've got strep throat," you rasp. Out come the cotton swab and the culture slide. She swipes the swab across the nether reaches of your throat. You gag. Depending on her stance on the use of antibiotics, the doctor may delay prescribing them until she gets the results of the throat culture. But when she gets those results, she will have a clear diagnosis. You either do or do not have strep throat.

Because there is no culture, no blood or urine test, no EKG or biopsy that specifically can diagnose bipolar disorder, you might wonder how your doctors arrived at that diagnosis. Like many psychiatric disorders, bipolar disorder can be difficult to diagnose. My own experience and reading about others illustrates that getting a correct diagnosis might only happen after

. . . getting a correct diagnosis might only happen after visiting multiple doctors and getting wrongly diagnosed . . .

visiting multiple doctors and getting wrongly diagnosed as having thyroid condition, Epstein-Barr, schizophrenia, attention-deficit hyperactivity disorder, or some other condition.

For many years, doctors have tried to refine and clarify the guidelines they use to diagnose psychiatric disorders. One standard set of guidelines is published in the American Psychiatric Association's *Diagnostic and Statistical Manual of Mental Disorders.* Now in its fourth edition (since 1994), it is called the *DSM-IV* for short, and there is also a *DSM-IV-TR* or text revision, from 2000. Something of a road map for mental health professionals, the *DSM-IV* attempts to guide them toward an appropriate diagnosis by identifying for them the signs and symptoms that tend to characterize a specific illness. By listening to patients' descriptions of their own experiences ("I'm hearing voices," "I can't eat," "I can't sleep") and by observing their behavior, professionals can evaluate the patient's information according to the *DSM-IV*'s definitions (called "criteria") of a given illness and its symptoms, and then arrive at a formal diagnosis. Often, the criteria for a certain mental illness will include a list of specific symptoms or indications; the patient need not have experienced *all* of these symptoms to be diagnosed as having that mental illness—only a certain set number. But as I noted earlier, the experience of a given mental illness varies from one person to the next, and this variation is one of the reasons mental illness can be so difficult to diagnose.

What is bipolar disorder? It is many things, but at its most basic, it is a chemical imbalance in the brain that can result in such outward symptoms as crippling depression, uncontrollable mania, and even psychosis. In a more clinical sense, bipolar disorder is the name that the *DSM-IV* currently attaches to certain clusters of symptoms (the mania, depression, and so on) that change in predictable patterns and occur in enough people often enough to be identifiable as part of a discrete (meaning distinct from others) condition. It belongs to a larger classification of illnesses called "mood disorders" or "affective disorders." What a condition is called matters because it determines the body of scholarship that tells doctors about available treatments and their rates of success. Some treatments are more successful than others; some things work for one condition but not for another; some drugs that are useful in treating one disorder can be harmful in treating another. (On one level, I don't care what they call it as long as they can find effective ways to eliminate or minimize the racing of my mind that occurs in one phase of this condition and the congealing of my ability to think and function that characterizes the other.) Lithium and Depakote, the brand name for the mood stabilizer valproic acid, are medications of first resort for bipolar disorder.

The Different Types of Bipolar Disorder

Bipolar disorder is divided into two types: bipolar I and bipolar II. Bipolar I is characterized by severe mania and severe depression. Think of it as a rocking chair that rocks forward and back sharply or a roller coaster that ascends and then descends through comparable lengths of track. The more common type, bipolar II, has depressions as deep as those of bipolar I, but less severe manias known as *hypomanias*. This rocking chair rocks

The more common type, bipolar II, has depressions as deep as those of bipolar I, but less severe manias known as hypomanias.

slightly forward but all the way back. If someone with bipolar II is hospitalized, it will probably be for the risk of suicide associated with depression, not for hypomania. I fall into the less common type, bipolar I.

Those with *cyclothymia* swing from hypomania to mild depression. Since neither mood is severe, this condition rarely requires hospitalization. When the swings of full-blown mania and major depression alternate more than four times a year, it is known as rapid cycling. The swings between states sometimes happen within the same day and are called ultra-rapid cycling. About 10% to 15% of those with manic depression experience rapid cycling. Most are women. Rapid cycling is disorienting, difficult to treat, and often requires hospitalization. Some describe it as the "yo-yo" of mood shifts.

Hypomania lies somewhere between a euthymic (normal) state and a full-blown mania; this seductive state is enjoyable and productive. Remember the Sirens from classical mythology? Their song was enticing, but become entranced by it and you are lost. Hypomania is a siren song. When you are hypomanic, you love life and feel good about yourself. People want to be around you. You lose inhibition and gain confidence, but not enough to get into the sort of serious trouble that characterizes psychoses. You don't feel just healthy, but *extremely* healthy and from that perspective can easily convince yourself that you no longer need medication. That conclusion is among the rocks at the end of a journey toward the sirens' song. Full-blown mania is another of the reefs into which you can crash.

In my case, manias are always followed by depressions or mixed states. The longer I stay energized, the deeper the depression afterward. For me, a rough proportion of time spent manic to the resulting depression is at least one to three. Recognizing signs of cycling and getting prompt treatment minimizes suffering.

There is also something called *unipolar mania,* which is the experience of mania without depression. In September 2002 one medical journal confirmed that about 16% of people with bipolar I experience unipolar mania.

The Symptoms of Bipolar Disorder

Mania: High Energy and Mood

The hallmarks of mania for me are racing thoughts and talking a mile a minute. According to the *DSM-IV-TR,* a diagnosis of mania is made when there is "a distinct period of abnormally and persistently elevated, expansive, or irritable mood." This period must last at least one week. Three (or more) of the following symptoms have persisted and have been present to a significant degree:

- An inflated self-esteem or grandiosity
- Decreased need for sleep (e.g., feels rested after only three hours of sleep)
- More talkative than usual or pressure to keep talking
- Flight of ideas or subjective experience that thoughts are racing
- Distractability (i.e., attention too easily drawn to unimportant or irrelevant external stimuli)
- Increase in goal-directed activity (either socially, at work or school, or sexually) or psychomotor agitation
- Excessive involvement in pleasurable activities that have a high potential for painful consequences (e.g., engaging in unrestrained buying sprees, sexual indiscretions, or foolish business investments).

Furthermore, for a diagnosis of mania, there should be no mixed state, no overactive thyroid (hyperthyroidism), and no drug abuse (with which mania is often mistaken). The *DSM-IV* adds that mania is an appropriate diagnosis if a hospitalization is required, even if the symptoms have lasted for less than one week, and it is not deemed bipolar I if the episode was caused by medication, electroconvulsive therapy (ECT), or light therapy.

. . . *mania is an intoxicatingly fun personal party, but in the long run it is painfully destructive.*

In short, mania is an intoxicatingly fun personal party, but in the long run it is painfully destructive. The reckless driving, lavish spending, unsafe sex, drug abuse, and other dangerous symptoms that it might trigger can be followed by unhealthy consequences, including personal injury, damage to personal relationships, a depression, mixed state, or psychotic episode, and the possibility of ending one's life by suicide.

In the 1920s, German psychiatrist Emil Kraepelin, the guru of the manic-depressive classification, described mania as "the incapacity to carry out consistently a definite series of thoughts, to work out steadily and logically and to set in order given ideas, also the fickleness of interest and the sudden and abrupt jumping from one subject to another." He added that a manic patient cannot be "convinced of the real nature of his state. He feels himself healthier and more capable than ever (and) has a colossal energy for work." Kraepelin's work laid the foundation for the modern study of bipolar disorder.

Mania can include racing thoughts, distractibility, elevated self-esteem, talkativeness, and a decreased need for sleep. When experiencing mania, I also lose the ability to think from other people's perspectives. My mind seems to be shutting down, taking with it my capacity to think, decide, interpret, and act on my own conclusions.

The following metaphors that people who are in a manic state use to capture the experience suggest exhilaration, speed, and lack of control: a racing engine, a speeding train, a comet, being painted in every color of the palette onto a canvas of glowing yellow, seeing the world through a kaleidoscope.

Most people with bipolar disorder have a combination of changes in both mood and energy. Luckily, not all of us become psychotic when we're manic. One reason I committed to continue medication and psychotherapy treatment is that I don't ever want to experience psychosis again.

Mania can be exasperating. I remember trying to think my way out of thinking too much and, when I failed, becoming agitated and angry. I think cessation of thought is impossible when you're manic. In her 1995 memoir *An Unquiet Mind*, psychiatry professor Kay Redfield Jamison describes one of her manias as "a neuronal pileup on the highways of my brain, and the more I tried to slow down my thinking the more I became aware I couldn't. My enthusiasms were going into overdrive as well, although there often was some underlying thread of logic in what I was doing." It's common to start but not to finish projects when you're manic. Your words and hands can't keep up with your racing ideas.

Another telltale sign of mania is excessive money spending. "I must have spent far more than thirty thousand dollars during my two major manic episodes," notes Jamison, "and God only knows how much more during my frequent milder manias." She describes a laundry list of frivolous items she bought on a whim with credit. I, too, find myself spending more when I'm manic. My reliance on cash rather than credit saves me from crushing debt.

> ## How Many Americans
> ## with Bipolar Disorder Are There?
>
> It is hard to estimate how many people have bipolar disorder, but one 2002 source claims that roughly 0.85% or 1.9 million adults (aged 15 and over) in the United States probably have bipolar I or bipolar II disorder. In males, the first episode of bipolar disorder is more likely to be mania than depression. In females, the opposite is true. For reasons that are unclear, in both Europe and the United States, bipolar disorder is more likely to be found among wealthier and better educated families; the reverse is true of schizophrenia. This is not totally attributable to the tendency of psychiatrists to diagnose those of lower socioeconomic status with schizophrenia.

Depression: The Lows

My own hallmark of depression is being physically still and talking very little because I have no energy or motivation. The *DSM-IV-TR* recommends a diagnosis of depression to be made when the person is experiencing either (1) depressed mood or (2) loss of interest or pleasure. The symptoms should be causing "clinically significant distress or impairment in social, occupational, or other areas of functioning" and should not be due "to the direct physiological effects of a substance or a general medical condition," such as an underactive thyroid (hypothyroidism). A *DSM-IV-TR* diagnosis of depression also requires that "five (or more) of the following symptoms have been present during the same two-week period and represent a change from previous functioning":

- Depressed mood most of the day, nearly every day

- Markedly diminished interest or pleasure in all, or almost all, activities

- Significant weight loss (not due to dieting) or weight gain, or decrease or increase in appetite nearly every day

- Insomnia or excessive sleeping (hypersomnia) nearly every day

- Behavior that seems overly keyed up or slowed down

- Fatigue or loss of energy nearly every day

- Feelings of worthlessness or excessive or inappropriate guilt (may be delusional) nearly every day

- Diminished ability to think or concentrate, or indecisiveness

Also symptomatic of depression are recurrent thoughts of death, recurrent suicidal thinking with or without a specific plan, or a suicide attempt. A diagnosis of depression has to meet many criteria, including that the symptoms are not better accounted for by bereavement (for example, sadness after the loss of a loved one).

A psychiatrist's checklist for evaluating depression includes dysphoric (unhappy) mood, self-deprecation, aggressive behavior, sleep disturbance or sleep complaints, changes in school performance or in attitudes toward school, diminished sociability, loss of usual energy, and change in appetite or weight. Translated into English, the psychiatrist expects a person who is depressed to feel unhappy, worthless, hostile, tired, and uninterested in loved ones and often preferring to spend time alone. Some people who are depressed wake up and can't fall back to

. . . the psychiatrist expects a person who is depressed to feel unhappy, worthless, hostile, tired, and uninterested in loved ones and often preferring to spend time alone.

sleep, some can't get out of bed. Some experience their depressive symptoms more intensely in the morning and as the day progresses feel some relief by evening. Others may experience the exact opposite pattern.

Put differently, the depressions of bipolar disorder are characterized by sadness, low self-esteem, and loss of interest in activities. Other signs of depression are guilt, insomnia, and difficulty concentrating and coming up with ideas. For the depressed person, speaking is work, not pleasure. One's libido withers. I don't feel I'm attractive to anyone when I'm depressed. That response to these symptoms seems sensible. Feeling attractive isn't consistent with feeling unhappy, disinterested, tired, and worthless.

The metaphors those who are depressed use to describe their experiences are often passive, dark, deep, and dangerous: falling down a well, dropping into a bottomless pit, sliding down an endless chute, being sucked into a black hole, being painted in shades of gray onto a gray canvas, seeing the world through darkened glasses, existing in a world of shadows.

Feeling blue and being depressed are different. As Norman Endler wrote in his 1982 book, *Holiday of Darkness: A Psychologist's Personal Journey Out of His Depression,* the illness "pervades a person's life and seriously interferes with day-to-day functioning." To qualify as a depression, a mood state must be intense, long-lived, and characterized by agitated or retarded motor behavior, including slow or slurred speech. Where some people with bipolar who are depressed see drops in sleep and appetite, others reverse this pattern and sleep and eat more than they usually do. In his 1990 memoir *Darkness Visible,* the author William Styron described his own severe depression by saying, "All sense of hope had vanished, along with the idea of a futurity; my brain, in thrall to its outlaw hormones, had become less an organ of thought than an instrument registering, minute by minute, varying degrees of its own suffering."

Kraepelin noted that "the eye becomes dull." Norman Endler's wife reports that she could see the depression in his eyes. My friends say the same thing. They also can look at a photo of me and judge whether I was depressed at the time it was taken. When depressed I walk hunched over and sit in a slouch.

How desperate does depression make a person? Kay Redfield Jamison describes it in *An Unquiet Mind* as "a pitiless, unrelenting pain that affords no window of hope, no alternative to a grim and brackish existence, and no respite from the cold undercurrents of thought and feeling that dominate the horribly restless nights of despair."

Mixed State: Manic Mind, Depressed Body

My first psychiatrist, Dr. Gottstein, had a name for why, at the age of 17, I felt so awful. The unwelcome houseguest is called the *mixed state*, and mine liked to linger. Bipolar disorder manifests itself in many mood and energy combinations. There are shallow depressions and manias lasting a few weeks and then at other points deep depressions and manias lasting longer. The so-called mixed state occurs when manic and depressive traits occur in combination. In fact, research in 2005 reported that up to 40% of admissions to hospitals for bipolar disorder were characterized by mixed states. I find mixed states the most uncomfortable aspect of bipolar disorder for myself in part because they are hard to escape. However, the research says the hardest mood state to break is a severe depression.

The so-called mixed state occurs when manic and depressive traits occur in combination.

Mixed states are hard to explain because people without bipolar disorder probably never feel this bad in quite the same way. If you couldn't sleep for days, had a never-ending stream of racing thoughts you *really* didn't want to think about, and your body felt like a hollow achy husk run over by a caravan of trucks, you'd be on your way to feeling this miserable. My metaphors don't work well enough to express how terrible I feel during these mixed states.

Diagnosing Bipolar Disorder: A Close-Up of the Difficulties

The symptoms of bipolar disorder are not identical from person to person. Because of that and because a doctor's knowledge of what an individual is experiencing is largely based on what that person is able to relate, the diagnosis of one doctor may differ from that of another. In addition, the *DSM-IV* says that the symptoms "should represent a change from previous functioning." But part of what complicates the process of determining what it is we are experiencing is the fact that those evaluating us don't know what we are like ordinarily. Some people have more energy than others; some are more pessimistic than others. The diagnosticians try to determine how, if at all, the behaviors, thoughts, and moods we are experiencing differ from our norms or our baseline personalities. To do so, they have to rely on our reports and those of our families to determine whether what might be a change for someone else is actually the status quo for us. Another aspect of this medical illness is that its onset can be insidious, with symptoms evolving over time, which presents a diagnostic challenge for the physician, families, and the person suffering from the illness.

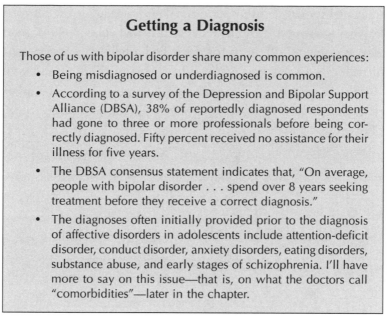

Getting a Diagnosis

Those of us with bipolar disorder share many common experiences:

- Being misdiagnosed or underdiagnosed is common.
- According to a survey of the Depression and Bipolar Support Alliance (DBSA), 38% of reportedly diagnosed respondents had gone to three or more professionals before being correctly diagnosed. Fifty percent received no assistance for their illness for five years.
- The DBSA consensus statement indicates that, "On average, people with bipolar disorder . . . spend over 8 years seeking treatment before they receive a correct diagnosis."
- The diagnoses often initially provided prior to the diagnosis of affective disorders in adolescents include attention-deficit disorder, conduct disorder, anxiety disorders, eating disorders, substance abuse, and early stages of schizophrenia. I'll have more to say on this issue—that is, on what the doctors call "comorbidities"—later in the chapter.

There's also the problem with the way our society views certain types of experience. Some scholars believe that mental health/mental illness, sane/insane, and normal/abnormal are simply value-laden words that assume that one is the opposite of the other and that one is desirable and the other is not. Others believe that the two are not opposites, but rather categories on a continuum. This is an increasingly common point of view. As the then–U.S. Surgeon General Dr. David Satcher stated in 1999: "[M]ental health' and 'mental illness' are not polar opposites but may be thought of as points on a continuum. . . . Considering health and illness as points along a continuum helps one appreciate that neither state exists in pure isolation from the other."

In addition, before buying into the notion that some set of behaviors is normal and some other set abnormal, it is important to ask what notion of "normal" is at play in the *DSM-IV* if by its definitions between one-third and one-half of the population is abnormal. The *DSM-IV*, which was published in 1994, lists more than 300 mental disorders. In the face of that number, who's actually "normal"?

It is difficult to draw a line that separates those on the mentally ill continuum who need treatment and those who don't because of a muddled middle of those who function but could cope better with treatment. We are ultimately better served if this debate can be resolved, and a good first step would be in the area of "health insurance parity"—that is, health coverage that pays the same for the treatment of mental illness as for the treatment of physical illness.

> It is difficult to draw a line that separates those on the mentally ill continuum who need treatment and those who don't . . .

Another good step would be a true national public health plan that would provide voluntary preventive mental health checks and, when indicated, appropriate treatment. Just like when you go to the dentist and get fluoride treatment to prevent cavities or to the pediatrician for "well baby" visits.

What "Causes" Bipolar Disorder?

Something in the Brain?

Some researchers make a distinction between functional and biological illness. Functional disorders are problems in living—in interacting with others and performing the basic tasks required for everyday life, such as taking care of one's daily needs sufficiently, holding down a job, and avoiding harmful behaviors. Biological disorders are assumed to be physically based—

These paintings are by people who have or may have had bipolar disorder.

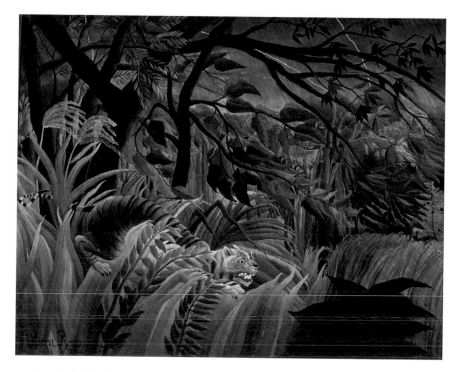

Tropical Thunderstorm with a Tiger (Surprised!),
by French artist Henri Rousseau (1844–1910)
National Gallery, London/Erich Lessing/Art Resource, New York

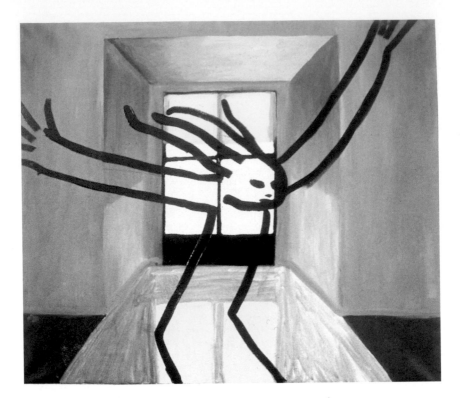

Cry in the Empty Room, by contemporary
American artist Meghan Caughey
The Bipol Art Project: www.bipol-art.de;
© *Meghan Caughey*

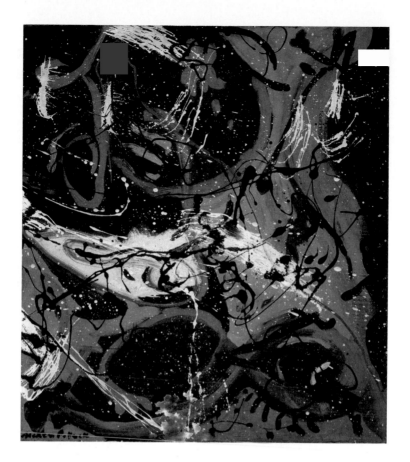

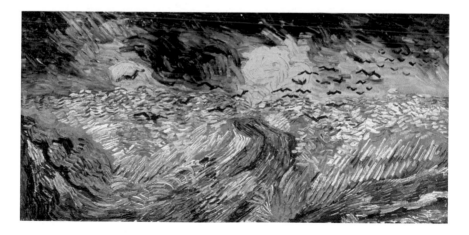

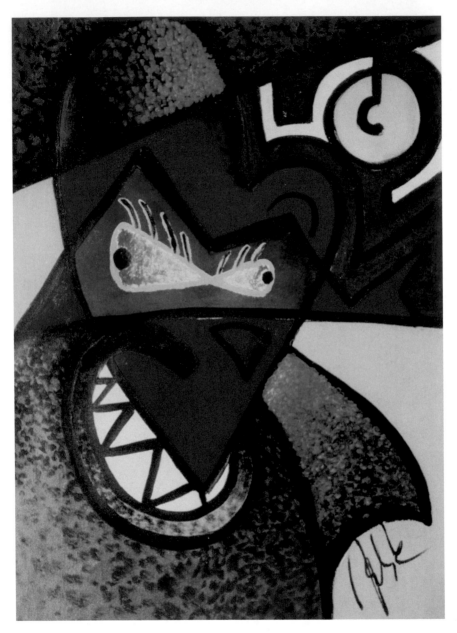

Time Machine, by contemporary German artist Alexander Zalik
The Bipol Art Project: www.bipol-art.de

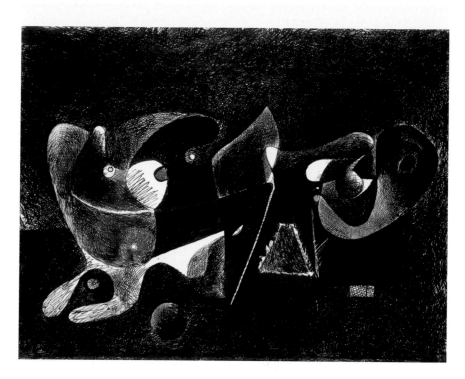

Nighttime, Enigma, and Nostalgia, by Armenian-born American artist
Arshile Gorky (1904–1948)
*Ailsa Mellon Bruce Fund and Andrew W. Mellon Fund, image © 2005
Board of Trustees, National Gallery of Art, Washington, DC.*
© 2006 Artists Rights Society (ARS), New York

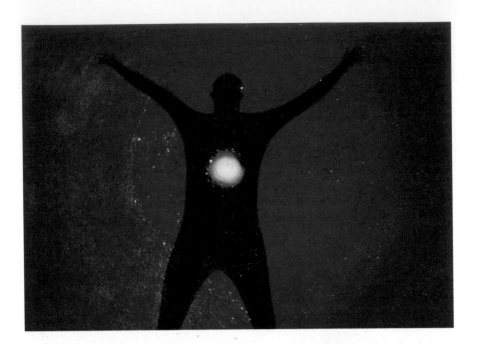

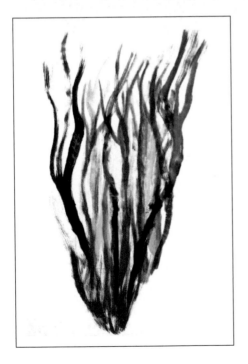

Above: Mania,
by contemporary
German artist Tobias Fritz
The Bipol Art Project:
www.bipol-art.de

Left: Crash, by
contemporary German
artist Michael Werner
The Bipol Art Project:
www.bipol-art.de

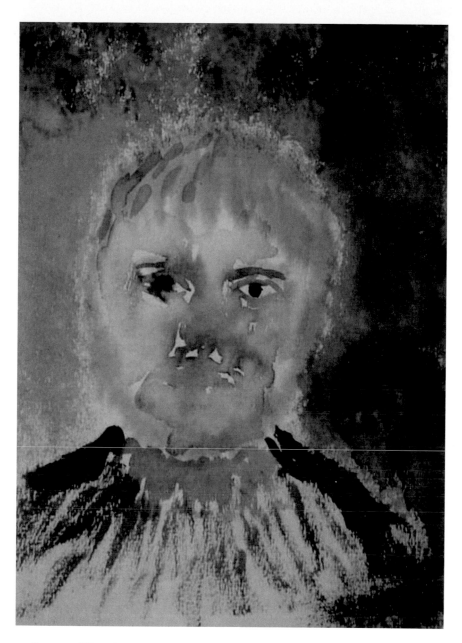

Become Silent, by contemporary German artist Michael Werner
The Bipol Art Project: www.bipol-art.de

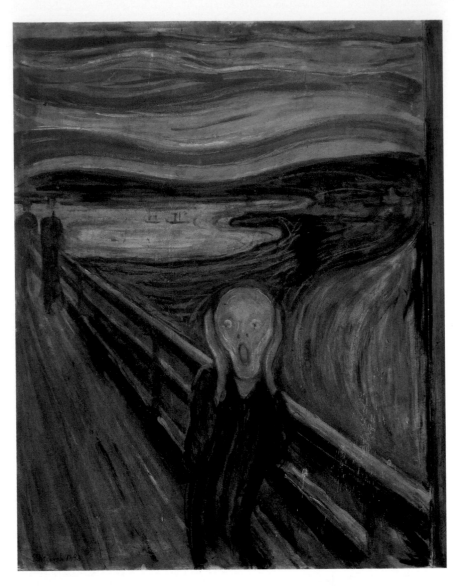

The Scream, by Norwegian artist Edvard Munch (1863–1944)
Erich Lessing/Art Resource, New York. © 2006 The Munch Museum/The Munch Ellingsen Group/Artists Rights Society (ARS), New York

examples would be heart disease or cancer. When bipolar disorder proved unresponsive to such interventions as talk therapy (which would address a functional disorder) and did respond to lithium, many said, "Aha, wrong classification!" and shifted it from the "functional" group to the "biological" one (because such disorders respond to medication intervention).

There are many theories pointing to the physiological nature of bipolar disorder, among them the theory that the condition is characterized by the slowing down or speeding up of communications between the nerve cells in the brain. Psychological expression of these biochemical changes includes mood and energy swings, delusions, and both euphoria and dysphoria (which is malaise, vexation, a generalized state of feeling unwell or unhappy). Some theorize that bipolar disorder may manifest itself when those who are predisposed to having the illness experience a "trigger" in their environment. This predisposition is possibly created by an individual's genetic framework. This means that something in a person's unique internal makeup—say, the way one's brain is wired—may be upset by something stressful in the person's surroundings. For me, the stress of the move to Hawaii is an example of the kind of the potential stressful environmental triggers these theorists mean.

But the truth is that although certain parts of the brain (the amygdala, for instance) have recently been identified as being a different size in youth with bipolar disorder, for the moment researchers still don't know why bipolar disorder happens or how to prevent it from happening.

Something in the Genes?

The most consistent "risk factor" for bipolar disorder—that is, the characteristic that most often increases someone's chances of

The most consistent "risk factor" . . . is family history.

developing the illness—is family history. Studies of twins, for example, suggest that it is probably genetic, meaning that if one identical twin has bipolar disorder, the other is more likely than a non-twin to experience it as well. Other interesting points:

- Twelve percent of the first-degree relatives (sisters, brothers, parents, and first cousins) of those with manic depression suffer from major depression.

- The Depression and Bipolar Support Alliance wrote in 2005 that "Bipolar disorder is more likely to affect the children of parents who have the disorder. When one parent has bipolar disorder, the risk to each child is estimated to be 15–30%. When both parents have bipolar disorder, the risk increases to 50–75%."

- Women whose close relatives have mood disorders are 2.4 times as likely as those without that genetic link to react to a stressful situation by becoming manic or depressed.

- Overall, according to one 1998 handbook for medical professionals, "[f]rom 80–90% of bipolar patients have a parent, sibling, or child with a mood disorder."

Researchers now think that bipolar disorder probably involves multiple genes. The good news is that as with other illnesses, having a particular genetic variant doesn't automatically mean you'll develop the condition. For example, the gene may be modified by other variations in the person's genetic makeup. Furthermore, the fact that the onset of bipolar disorder is so unpredictable indicates that environmental factors

When Does Bipolar Disorder Occur, How Often, and for How Long?

- The onset of bipolar disorder can occur in the teenage years. One source stated in 1999 that the "average age of onset for manic-depression bipolar illness is about seventeen or eighteen."

- Ninety-five percent of those with the condition experience more than one episode. One study found that the number of episodes in a lifetime ranged from 2 to more than 30. Forty-two percent had more than ten episodes with the median number being nine, with "episode" defined as a time period characterized by a mania or depression.

- If it is untreated, according to one report by Kay Redfield Jamison in 1999, "mania lasts from one to three months, and bipolar depression, if left untreated, will last for at least six to nine months on average. . . . Later in life, the intervals between episodes may diminish so markedly that the disease looks like a chronic illness."

(e.g., stressful life events) also play a major role in this disease, although there is much more to learn about the extent to which this may be true.

Can Other Conditions Occur with Bipolar Disorder?

Yes, bipolar disorder does often exist side by side with other emotional and behavioral disorders, which can make diagnosis and treatment more complicated. Some of these "comorbid conditions," as they're called, include the following:

- **Attention-deficit hyperactivity disorder** (ADHD), in which symptoms have to be present before age seven, is characterized by hyperactivity, inattention, or both, plus impulsiveness. Although mania by itself does occur in children, it is very rare. In some, a severe form of ADHD may be an early manifestation of the emerging mania of bipolar I disorder. In other instances, the two seem to co-exist. Given the many similarities, the potential for mis-diagnosis is high, but most experts agree that there are significant distinctions between the two. For example, dangerous behavior by an adolescent with bipolar disor-der often seems to be impulsive decision making based on distorted thinking, while the same behavior by a teen with ADHD is more typically caused by general inattentive-ness and impulsiveness. A complex blend of the two be-havior patterns may be seen in adolescents who have both bipolar disorder and ADHD at once. Scientists are cur-rently conducting clinical research involving children and adolescents struggling with these symptoms to tease out the relationship between these illnesses.

- **Anxiety disorders** One in five of those with bipolar disor-der will also have a panic disorder.

- **Substance abuse** According to a study in 1994, 52% of teenagers who experienced bipolar disorder before age 20 had drug or alcohol abuse problems. The National Insti-tute of Mental Health reported in 2001 that a sign of mania includes abusing drugs, including alcohol, cocaine, and sleeping pills.

- **Conduct disorder** Characterized by extreme difficulty fol-lowing the rules or behaving in a socially acceptable way. As with ADHD, there is some symptom overlap between conduct disorder and bipolar disorder. One differentiat-ing factor is the presence of guilt. Kids with bipolar disorder often feel guilty when there's no reason to feel this way, while those with conduct disorder usually feel no remorse when they've done something wrong.

- **Oppositional defiant disorder** Characterized by a long-lasting pattern of defiance, uncooperativeness, and hostility toward authority figures, including parents. Adolescents with either bipolar disorder or oppositional defiant disorder can appear quite irritable, surly, aggressive, and prone to temper tantrums. In addition, the grandiose beliefs of mania often look a lot like defiance to adults, since manic teenagers who are convinced of their own superior abilities or superhuman powers may not feel as if they need to listen to anyone else. As with ADHD and conduct disorder, getting a correct diagnosis depends on finding an experienced professional who can tell whether the problem is really bipolar disorder, oppositional defiant disorder, or both.

The Dangers of Doing Nothing

It is hard to admit that you have problems or that you cannot handle them without help. But the truth is that denying your problems, or thinking they'll just go away with time, or facing them but trying to deal with them by yourself, is not a viable answer. You need to seek treatment from a qualified mental health professional. Otherwise, you face an uphill battle that you likely won't win. People with untreated mood disorders (bipolar or major depression) are more likely to do poorly in school, to abuse substances, and to engage in risky behaviors such as reckless driving. According to the Centers for Disease

Control and Prevention in 2001, unintentional injuries, most of which are due to car accidents, are the number one killer of young Americans ages 15 to 24. Suicide is also a major risk. In fact, the suicide risk for those with bipolar disorder is more than 20 times higher than those without it, and those with untreated mental disorders are at the highest risk for suicide. If you are having suicidal thoughts or planning suicide, tell a parent or responsible adult friend and get medical help immediately. The crisis numbers 1-800-SUICIDE or 911 are valuable resources in an emergency.

If you are having suicidal thoughts or planning suicide, tell a parent or responsible adult friend and get medical help immediately.

The Bottom Line

What's the bottom line? Although there is not yet a reliable test to confirm its presence, we do know when bipolar disorder is likely to appear and what some of its patterns are. Despite the fact that they have not isolated its causes, doctors have found treatments that work reasonably well for many people much of the time. They have also developed a set of guidelines that help manage the condition. If you were misdiagnosed before finding the doctors who recognized the condition, you've got a lot of company. Our latest episode will probably not be our last, but there are things that we can do to cut the odds in our favor. These treatments are the subjects of the following chapters.

Chapter Four

Getting Help

Endure, and preserve yourselves for better things.

–Virgil, *Aeneid*

I t is important for people with bipolar disorder to have quality health care, but what does this entail? Although there are
very few child or adolescent psychiatrists in the United States,
a good way to find one who specializes in pediatric bipolar
disorder is by getting a referral from your pediatrician or family practitioner, contacting a teaching hospital associated with
a medical school, or using the American Academy of Child
and Adolescent Psychiatry's referral directory (see the Resources
section at the end of this book). For young people over 18,
however, an adult psychiatrist may be preferred and indeed is
easier to find, given that there are many more adult psychiatrists in the country.

I live in a major city and have health care benefits, so I have
been fortunate enough to have a choice of mental health care
providers. Initially my general practitioner referred me to a child
psychiatrist, and years later, when I was no longer a minor, I
transferred to an adult psychiatrist. I was still getting sick during
college, so I went to a third psychiatrist to help me better manage my disorder. When he stopped practicing, he referred me to
a highly experienced psychiatrist who has kept me functioning

well and out of the hospital ever since. In other words, persistence in finding the right treatment provider pays off.

But what are the treatments available to help you with bipolar disorder? This chapter is presented as a brief, introductory catalog of the types of treatments you may encounter.

Medication

Psychopharmacological treatment (taking medication) is an essential part of treating bipolar disorder. Medications are prescribed by a psychiatrist or other medical professional (in some states, clinical psychologists and advanced nurse practitioners may prescribe as well). Lithium, Depakote, and other mood stabilizers are the most commonly used medications for people with the illness.

Mood Stabilizers

LITHIUM

Although it is an element naturally found in ancient alkaline spring water, lithium's antimanic properties were not discovered until 1948, when an Australian psychiatrist named John Cade did so accidentally while conducting experiments on guinea pigs. Lithium was later tested on humans, and in the early 1970s the U.S. Food and Drug Administration (FDA) approved lithium's use in people. Today it is the longest-tested mood stabilizer for the treatment of bipolar disorder. As an added bonus, some evidence shows that patients who take lithium may be less likely to kill themselves. The bad news is that 42% to 64% of adults do not respond to it. Similarly, about half of young people respond to it and half don't. And as in all medications, lithium does have some unpleasant side effects. Most common are tremors, weight gain, and drowsiness. There is a therapeutic blood level for lithium treatment, and too much lithium in the blood can be toxic. Individuals treated with lithium will need regular blood monitoring not only for their lithium level but also for additional effects that chronic lithium treatment can lead to, such as hypothyroidism and change in kidney function. If you take lithium, it is important to drink plenty of water, especially in summer when perspiration can lead to an increased concentration of lithium in your blood.

If you take lithium, it is important to drink plenty of water.

Anticonvulsants

Anticonvulsant medications were initially used to treat epilepsy by preventing seizures, and now we know that valproic acid (Depakote) and carbamazepine (Tegretol), both anticonvulsants, can work as mood stabilizers for bipolar disorder as well. Since many cannot tolerate or benefit from lithium, anticonvulsants offer additional options for treating bipolar disorder. Like lithium, carbamazepine and valproic acid users need ongoing monitoring of blood levels and other laboratory tests to watch for the development of blood and/or liver changes that can occur with chronic treatment with these medications. Commonly occurring side effects of carbamazepine are clumsiness, drowsiness, dizziness, and vomiting. For valproic acid, side effects include nausea, headaches, double vision, dizziness, anxiety, and confusion. Women need to be especially concerned about the benefits and risks of using these medications if they plan on becoming pregnant and/or want to breastfeed. In one study from 2002, for example, some menstrual and ovarian abnormalities were reported in women who had epilepsy and took valproic acid.

A Special Note about Medication for Women with Bipolar Disorder

This is not meant to scare but to educate: Using lithium, especially in the first trimester of a woman's pregnancy, has been linked to cases of congenital malformations and other serious complications in the fetus. Furthermore, mothers who take lithium and breastfeed can cause lithium toxicity in their child. In general, using valproic acid or carbamazepine while pregnant can make congenital anomalies two to three time more likely. Valproic acid has been judged safe to use while breastfeeding, but doctors say infants whose mothers used carbamazepine should be carefully monitored. It is crucial to work with your doctor closely and carefully on this issue. Researchers point out that choosing a medication wisely, using the minimum effective dose, using only one drug, and limiting the duration the drug is taken all can help make the combination of being bipolar and using medication while pregnant or breastfeeding safer.

Lamotrigine (Lamictal), another anticonvulsant, is the first FDA-approved therapy since lithium for maintenance treatment of bipolar I. It appears to be effective at alleviating bipolar depression, while lithium traditionally has been described as best at reducing manias. Side effects include nausea, insomnia, and mild rashes that usually resolve themselves on their own. However, there appears to be an increased risk in adolescents taking Lamictal to develop a life-threatening rash called Stevens-Johnson syndrome. Although this is a rare event, as noted earlier in the book, I was one of the young people who did develop this side effect so seriously that it required hospitalization to manage. Most experts recommend starting lamotrigine slowly to help minimize any potential serious rashes.

Antidepressants

Antidepressants such as monoamine oxidase inhibitors (MAOIs) and tricyclics (TCAs) used to treat adult depression are not prescribed for children and adolescents. The MAOIs have dietary restrictions that physicians are concerned that adolescents would not follow, and the TCAs have been associated with cardiac sudden deaths. There are more modern antidepressants called SSRIs, or selective serotonin reuptake inhibitors, which became widely available in the 1980s and 1990s and work by increasing the amount of the neurotransmitter serotonin available to aid communication between neurons in the brain. These SSRIs include fluoxetine (Prozac), which is the only one approved for use in children and adolescents suffering from depression, paroxetine (Paxil), sertraline (Zoloft), and others. Bupropion (Wellbutrin) is called an atypical antidepressant because its means of acting on the brain is different from that of the other antidepressants.

There has been concern in recent years that treatment with antidepressants was causing suicidal thinking in some young people. In the late summer of 2004, the FDA released a study that suggested antidepressants with various mechanisms of action might increase the risk of suicidal thoughts and behaviors among children and adolescents. The following October, the FDA directed the makers of antidepressants to add to their product labels a "black box warning" about this risk and about the need for close supervision of young people who are prescribed such medications. This underscores the importance of careful monitoring by a mental health professional when you are taking these medications and the necessity of your being honest with your doctor about any suicidal thoughts. Also, you and your family should review with your prescribing physician all of the potential side effects that could occur with the particular medication you are taking. Most side effects are mild to moderate in nature and often resolve after several weeks of treatment. However, certain types of side effects, such as feeling increased agitation, irritability, and impulsivity, may be related to increased risk for suicidal thinking and/or behaviors. Another potential consequence of using antidepressants to treat bipolar depression includes triggering a manic episode; there can also be withdrawal symptoms from stopping the medication quickly. Be sure to honestly inform your physician about any changes in symptoms or new symptoms that you are experiencing, and tell your doctor if you plan on quitting a medication.

> *Be sure to honestly inform your physician about any changes in symptoms or new symptoms that you are experiencing . . .*

Antipsychotics

The treatments for mania and psychoses have improved greatly since the 1700s, when no useful treatments were available. In those days, the general public in one of our largest cities, Philadelphia, was charged admission to asylums so that they could heckle the mentally ill. But then, in the middle of the 20th century, there was a psychopharmacological revolution, and subsequent refinements to antipsychotic medication have allowed people with mania and/or psychosis to be brought down from that state and allowed to sleep and heal. One of these drugs is haloperidol (Haldol), an older generation antipsychotic with significant side effects. Though it can cloud the mind and make the joints stiff, my hospital ward gave it to me regularly into the 1990s, possibly to save money, even though some of its other side effects, such as tardive dyskinesia (facial twitches and worm-like movements of the tongue), can be irreversible. This risk is minimized with the newer, more costly atypical antipsychotic medications, such as clozapine (Clozaril), olanzapine (Zyprexa), quetiapine (Seroquel), risperidone (Risperdal), and ziprasidone (Geodon). There are also drugs that are used to complement the antipsychotics, such as Ativan (lorazepam), an antianxiety drug that can quickly relax you.

Haloperidol and the atypical antipsychotic risperidone are used to treat severe mental disorders, including ones with hallucinations and delusions. The newer atypical antipsychotics, such as olanzapine (Zyprexa) and clozapine (Clozaril), have side effects ranging from weight gain to high blood sugar to diabetes. Clozaril has the additional requirement of a weekly blood test in order to monitor for the occurrence of decreased white blood cell numbers.

Implications of Medication Therapy

It may seem strange that you should take medication when so much seems stacked up against doing so: It is expensive, you could be allergic to it, it may have troubling side effects, and most of what is known about many of the medications (except lithium) is from relatively short-term studies. Also, because the experience of manias and hypomanias can be so pleasurable, medicating them out of your life feels like the proverbial rain on your parade. But the reality is that if you're ill, you need help, which includes taking—and staying on—your meds, and there are ways that you can overcome or at least cope with the downside of having to be on them. You can, for example, find substantial cost savings if you are able to order your prescriptions online. You can be aware of and act quickly in the rare event of an allergic reaction to the medication you're on. You can counter weight gain through exercise, and there are even medications that can help manage other side effects, such as tremors. Also, you could try a different drug, one with the same mechanism of action, or one in a different group of medications, which may not lead to the side effects. There are newer medications with varying side effects available for treating different aspects of bipolar disorder—but remember that newer doesn't necessarily mean better. It can mean the meds are more expensive and that less is known about them because fewer trials have been run. Bottom line: Whatever medication you're prescribed, make sure you tell your doctor about any side effects you may be experiencing.

Why stay treated? Simply put, staying on your meds—what mental health professionals call "medication adherence"—is critical to getting well. People with treated mental illness are much less likely to kill themselves, for example, and a strong argument can be made that the benefits of appropriately prescribed and monitored medication in the treatment of bipolar disorder can outweigh the risks to the patient.

. . . a strong argument can be made that the benefits of appropriately prescribed and monitored medication in the treatment of bipolar disorder can outweigh the risks to the patient.

Attending "medication management sessions" can also help you to manage stress and prevent a return of symptoms that could lead to a hospital visit. In my own sessions, my psychiatrist and I team up to make sure that I am healthy and still on board with continuing my medication treatment. Also, we discuss and review my blood medication levels, and we talk about how I'm managing side effects and whether I'm minimizing life stress, getting to sleep regularly, and not abusing drugs. In other words, we make sure that I am managing my illness instead of allowing it to manage me.

Medication Tips

- Make taking your pills at the same time every day a ritual (when you eat breakfast, or brush your teeth) so that you don't miss a dose.
- Use weekly or monthly pill containers to store your medication and put them in a sealable plastic baggie when you travel so they don't wind up all over the bottom of your bag or suitcase.
- Put your medication in your carry-on baggage when you travel so you don't lose your meds if your checked bags are misplaced.
- When you get new medication, use the older medication first as long as it is not expired.
- Mark on your calendar when you have to order more meds or get new prescriptions well in advance.

Psychotherapy

For those of us with bipolar disorder, there is a proven benefit to receiving both medication and psychotherapy rather than one or the other (or neither). It can be hard to find appropriate psychotherapy, and while some general practitioners are comfortable prescribing antidepressants, they are not trained as therapists. But assuming you can find and pay for good therapy, here are some typical therapeutic approaches that you might encounter:

Cognitive-Behavioral Therapy

Cognitive-behavioral therapy (CBT) aims to correct negative patterns of thinking and behavior that may contribute to certain mental health disorders like depression. It is based in part on cognitive therapy (CT), which was created by Aaron Beck, an eminent psychiatrist at the University of Pennsylvania who is still a leading force in the effort to alleviate depression. Used primarily in adults, CT teaches the patient how to modify negative thinking to reduce feelings of hopelessness and depression. In this therapy the patient learns how to employ many thinking skills, including how to overcome irrational thoughts and beliefs and to avoid overgeneralizing negative events. An example of irrational thinking for me was my assuming years ago that the young woman I had asked out on a date—and who told me she was busy on Friday night—hated me. CT teaches people to stop automatic negative thoughts and open their minds to other possibilities. Maybe she really was busy and would go out with me some other time. If I'd asked her out again and she said, "No, not now or ever!"—then what? Instead of being pessimistic or overgeneralizing that all women hate me, I could learn to use perspective. She is just one woman—there are many more who are better suited to my needs, personality, and talents, so I will keep on asking women out until I find one who will go out with me. (This is how I found my wife!) Cognitive therapy teaches people to stop negative thought patterns before they lead to hopelessness and spread to impulses with more dire consequences—such as using illegal drugs and contemplating suicide.

> Cognitive therapy teaches people to stop negative thought patterns before they lead to hopelessness and spread to impulses with more dire consequences . . .

Beck and his colleagues have been testing cognitive therapy on adults who are at a high risk of suicide (the homeless, heroin addicts, and the impoverished), and the results look promising. In August 2005, Beck and colleagues reported that their cognitive therapy program of only 8 to 10 sessions (traditionally it is 15) reduced suicide risk in their patients by half.

CBT combines cognitive therapy with what is called behavior therapy. The behavior therapy component involves increasing the number of planned positive activities the patient will participate in. For me it would be going to a fun restaurant with a friend or family member, seeing a funny movie, or working on home improvements. In other words, instead of watching TV by yourself and ruminating about how much life and certain people have hurt you, you make plans and stay busy with positive people. CBT combines the thinking skills from cognitive therapy to reduce problematic thinking with reevaluation and positive planned-participation skills to alleviate depression.

CBT has been demonstrated to be as effective as medication in treating adults diagnosed with moderate to severe major depression alone, contingent on the therapist's skill level. According to one medical textbook in 2005, CBT appears to be effective in the treatment of depression in adolescents as well, but is still being evaluated. The therapy has also been shown to be an effective complement to, rather than a replacement for, pharmacotherapy (medications) to treat bipolar disorder. In fact, studies suggest that the addition of CBT leads to improved medication adherence, fewer hospitalizations, and improved overall quality of life through better management of the illness.

Interpersonal Therapy

Another treatment for depression is interpersonal therapy (IPT). In adult IPT, communication and interaction skills are developed to handle four major "problem areas," including role transitions, grief, interpersonal deficits, and interpersonal disputes. IPT for adolescents covers areas such as separation from parents, authority and autonomy issues, peer pressure, and loss. The idea is that, while mood disorders may be caused by genetic or biological factors, their more severe episodes may be *triggered* by stressful or difficult interpersonal interactions. IPT seeks to use talk therapy to identify and address triggering interpersonal problems, and the patient is helped to develop interaction skills to resolve these problems.

Social Rhythm Therapy

Social rhythm therapy (SRT) is based on regulating your social interactions and your circadian rhythms. The idea here is that disrupted circadian rhythms (daily activity cycles lasting 24 hours) can trigger mood cycling, so SRT helps individuals with bipolar disorder keep their moods on a more even keel by regulating their basic biological processes, such as eating, sleeping, and exposure to sunlight.

Family Therapy

CBT, IPT, and other psychotherapies are most used in one-on-one sessions between a therapist and a client, but some of them may be used in group settings as well. Family therapy is one example, which involves bringing several members of a family together for therapy sessions. It can help families work together to identify and change the destructive patterns that may contribute to or arise from a teen's illness. It can also open lines of communication and teach everyone coping skills for dealing with that illness. Other possible goals include strengthening family bonds, improving empathy among family members, and reducing conflict in the home.

Indeed, stress and conflict at home can play a role in triggering mood episodes. A teen's manic behavior, in turn, can quickly ratchet up the stress and strain for everyone else. It's little surprise, then, that several studies of people who have recently been hospitalized for bipolar disorder have found that those who returned home to a stressful environment were at increased risk for relapse. By contrast, a study in 1990 indicated that by improving coping skills and reducing negative family behaviors, patients had less depression, better medication adherence, and fewer hospitalizations. The point is that a calmer home makes life more pleasant for everyone while reducing the relapse risk for the teen with bipolar disorder. Family therapy can help your family work together as a unit toward this goal.

. . . a calmer home makes life more pleasant for everyone while reducing the relapse risk for the teen with bipolar disorder.

What do I take away from these various psychotherapies? I have learned that I am healthiest when I use reframing and perspective to manage automatic negative thinking and when I am planning social activities. I focus on getting up and going to bed at the same time every day, on trying to eat meals at regular times, and on having a job that doesn't require too much travel across time zones so I can have regular sleep.

Cool Down: Defuse Now Before You Explode

Early on in my adventure with bipolar disorder, during my manic-ridden high school years, I would sometimes get into verbal confrontations with my parents that escalated into all-out fights. My psychiatrist suggested that in these instances, I could do damage control and defuse the situation by leaving the room and letting things "cool down." Cooling down worked for me, and it could work for other young people. If everyone knows about this plan ahead of time, they would take less offense at the young person leaving the danger zone. This technique prevents verbal spats from escalating into something uglier so that more peaceful, healing, and therapeutic communication can take place later.

Other Therapies

Traditional medications and therapies work in most patients, but there are options for non-responders as well.

Light Therapy

Light therapy—also called phototherapy—involves a regimen of daily exposure to very bright light from an artificial source. The intensity of the light is similar to that of early morning sunlight and many times brighter than that of normal indoor light fixtures. While light therapy is not the first line of defense for bipolar disorder, researchers now know that there is a link between sunlight and depression. Winter depression, or seasonal affective disorder (SAD), can be alleviated in dark months by using a light box to put artificial sunlight into our eyes. These light boxes can be bought without a prescription. The industry standard has been a 10,000 lux exposure for 30 minutes a day. The advantage of this system is that light is natural. One drawback, however, is that it can be inconvenient to sit in front of a light box for half an hour each day instead of sleeping or doing other things. In any case, it is important to discuss with your doctor if your present treatment is not working and you want to consider adding a treatment like light therapy for the depressive phase of your illness. (A smart alternative to promoting a light-filled environment is to try to face a window with southern exposure at work and at home, or, since this is not an option for most of us, take a walk outside each day to get some sun.)

Why is the sun so important? There is a gland in the middle of our brains called Aristotle's lantern or the pineal gland. Specifically, the absence of sunlight prompts the pineal gland to release melatonin, a drug that helps us sleep. A recent study has shown that sunlight, artificial or real, stimulates the gland, thereby changing and regulating our body's circadian (daily) rhythms.

Dark Therapy

An interesting pilot study published in 2005 suggests a benefit for rapid-cycling bipolar patients who start treating their mania within two weeks of its onset with dark therapy—that is, 14 hours of darkness and bed rest from 6 P.M. to 8 A.M. for three consecutive days. Their mania subsided faster, they required less antimanic medication, and they were discharged from the hospital earlier. Although encouraging, the study was only a pilot and further research with larger sample sizes is necessary to better understand what is going on.

Electroconvulsive Therapy

Electroconvulsive therapy (ECT) is a well-researched and common procedure for treating depression in people who don't respond to other therapies, and it shows definite improvement in 75% of cases. In ECT, a seizure is induced intentionally by introducing an electric current to the brain while the patient is under full anesthesia. Doctors originally used insulin to produce these seizures because they were found to alleviate depression, but broken bones and fractured teeth sometimes resulted from the convulsions. Now, ECT is used in conjunction with anesthesia and muscle relaxants in order to induce depression-easing seizure safely and effectively. Some short-term memory loss is the one major side effect, and there is a very small mortality rate, but this procedure has been clinically proven to alleviate depression.

ECT (poorly nicknamed "shock treatment") has an undeserved bad reputation promoted by films such as *One Flew Over*

ECT (poorly nicknamed "shock treatment") has an undeserved bad reputation promoted by films such as One Flew Over the Cuckoo's Nest. the Cuckoo's Nest. Also, by today's standards, it was misused in the past, but now it is safe, fast, and very effective. As Norman Endler points out, "What most people [who criticize ECT] don't realize is that the depression itself 'fogs up' a person's mental and perceptual abilities. . . . Depression dulls our perceptions and we can neither concentrate nor pay attention. . . . Because of this, effective treatment should commence immediately, be it ECT or drugs." ECT isn't the problem. The depression is.

Vagus Nerve Stimulation

Vagus nerve stimulation therapy (VNS) was pioneered for treating epilepsy, but in the summer of 2005, the FDA approved it for the treatment of chronic depression in those who are 18 years or older. In VNS a battery is implanted under the skin, and electrical stimulation flows into the brain via the vagus nerve in the neck. With its ability to elevate mood, this therapy gives hope to depressed non-responders who have exhausted all other scientific treatment options to heal their depression.

Transcranial Magnetic Stimulation

Transcranial magnetic stimulation (TMS) is an investigational therapy that creates a magnetic field around the patient's head to alter the brain chemistry. Testing is being conducted to find out how effective it really is at alleviating depression, reducing mania, and treating other psychiatric disorders. It is not yet approved for use by the general public.

Charting Your Mood and Energy

Here is a fun way to learn more about your mental health: To chart your moods, start by buying a yearlong calendar or obtain one for a small fee from the Depression and Bipolar Support Alliance (see the Resources section for the address). On each day that your mood is severely manic, color the day on the calendar red; if you feel somewhat manic, color it orange; if your mood is somewhat elevated, color it yellow; if you feel "normal," color it white; if somewhat depressed, blue; if moderately depressed, purple; and if severely depressed, black. Any day can include multiple colors.

Then, to chart the days, translate the colors into numbers and graph them: red +3, orange +2, yellow +1, white O, blue −1; purple −2, and black −3. This chart will help you determine whether there is a monthly, weekly, or daily pattern to your moods, whether you are predictably affected by the seasons, and how well your medication is working.

How to Handle Suicidal Thoughts

It bears repeating that if you feel like hurting yourself, you need to get help. Tell a friend, a parent, or other trusted adult. You or your family should call your doctor, a licensed therapist, or community health agency right away. In an emergency, call 1-800-SUICIDE or 911.

Unfortunately, because suicide is a taboo topic in American culture, we are taught not to share our thoughts and feelings about it. But talking about suicide doesn't cause people to become suicidal. In fact, talking about it is a crucial step toward getting help and feeling better. You want to find

Unfortunately, because suicide is a taboo topic in American culture, we are taught not to share our thoughts and feelings about it.

and stay with responsible people who will remind you that there are positive options for you and who will help you get assistance if needed.

Hospitalization

Outpatient psychiatric services (like the medications and therapies listed above) are an option for many young people, but there are some times when inpatient treatment is necessary, such as when someone

- poses a threat to himself or herself, or to others

- is behaving in a bizarre or destructive manner

- requires medication that must be closely monitored

- needs round-the-clock care to become stabilized

- has not improved in outpatient care

If you are going to be hospitalized, it is important to do everything you can to get into the best facility available that takes your insurance. I visited a ward a few years ago to see a friend who was suicidal and had been taken to the only facility in the area with available beds. Within minutes, I got an appreciation for how much better my old ward was run. My friend's nurses weren't enforcing rules that I had taken for granted when I was hospitalized, such as patients not touching or harassing other patients. While as described in the next chapter my own experiences in the psych ward were far from idyllic, and despite my disagreements with some of the staff, the ward was organized well enough to allow me to recover each time I visited.

Chapter Five

The Psychiatric Ward

[O]ne flew east, one flew west, one flew over the cuckoo's nest . . . goose swoops down and plucks you out.

—Ken Kesey, *One Flew Over the Cuckoo's Nest* (1962)

From Kitchen Floor to Emergency Door

When I was diagnosed at 15, my psychiatrist gave me his card and said I could call him at any hour. If I felt that it was an emergency, I could call in the middle of the night or on a weekend. I liked that he said, "If you feel it is an emergency," not "if it is an emergency." The determination was not someone else's. It was mine. If I felt that it was an emergency, then by definition it was an emergency. I put the card in my wallet.

If I felt that it was an emergency, then by definition it was an emergency.

When newly diagnosed I hadn't yet developed a sixth sense or a clear perspective about the disorder. The advantage of having been through any process is that you know the drill. As a result, the first time is the roughest. My first hospitalization occurred 18 months after diagnosis. I was a senior in high school at the time.

Mania was kicking into high gear. The mind race in my head was on. I felt as if I were simultaneously directing and starring in my own movie. My experiences were freaky, even for a 17-year-old tough guy who thought he could handle anything. That fall, at 3:30 A.M. in the middle of a work week, I called the number on the card and asked for Dr. Gottstein. The number on the card reached his "service"—medical jargon for a person who takes calls and relays messages to doctors.

A brusque male voice answering the phone loudly griped that it was 3:30 in the morning! Was I aware that if he relayed my message he'd awaken Dr. Gottstein? After cradling the phone, I folded into an origami-like ball on the kitchen floorboards and started to cry. Lying there, what coherence was left in my brain signaled a realization. If I thought this was an emergency, it was an emergency.

I redialed and declared to the voice that this was an emergency. Dr. Gottstein called back within a few minutes. The fact that he had called back promptly was reassuring. The call had obviously wakened him. His voice was more distant, the pace of his words slower than the usual back and forth in his office. But I recognized the voice, and our relationship clicked in. He asked me to describe my symptoms. After I had done so, he instructed me to go to the hospital ER. He would call to tell them I was coming.

Admission to the hospital that night was my first since birth, and that time I wasn't the one who had to handle the hassle of admission. Had I recognized the onset of mania, I could have avoided this new experience with a telephone call and a low dose of antipsychotic medication two and a half weeks earlier.

Thinking we knew where we were going and that we were following Dr. Gottstein's directions, my parents and I went to the wrong emergency room where we waited for five hours before I was mistakenly evaluated as a victim of child abuse, asked questions about sexual touching, and subjected to a humiliating examination by a young—and female—ER doctor.

Afterward, we realized that there are two emergency rooms near one another. That was why we could find no one who had heard from my doctor. I was in the wrong place being treated by the wrong person for the wrong problem at the wrong time. After finding the right emergency room, we waited another four hours until I was finally admitted.

During that four-hour period, I was transformed into someone whose name was "the patient" or "pt" in the medical notepads:

> Starting at age 12 [I was actually 11], the patient began experiencing episodes of hypomania lasting several months. The patient has had several episodes over the past year between episodes of hypomania, the patient became sick with mononucleosis, flu, etc. His first episode of depression was 1988, which lasted several weeks. The intensity of the manic episodes increased over the past few years. Around 18 months ago, the patient was started on Lithium and Clonopin to which he responded very well. However, the patient decided that he would like to try stopping his medications. The patient stopped taking the medications on his own about 8 months ago, although Dr. Gottstein had been speaking to him about stopping the medications. Roughly two months ago, the patient became symptomatic and Lithium was restarted.

Responding to questions about my medical and psychiatric history, I speak in monosyllables:

Do you feel comfortable with other people? "Yeah."
Do you feel someone is against you or may attempt to harm you? "No."
Do you hear voices? "No."
Do you have any strange thoughts? "Oh, sure."
Do you feel nervous or tense? "Hell, no."
Does your heart pound? "Oh, yeah. That's my problem—when I try
   to go to sleep. Bah bum bah bum."
Are you restless? "I don't have any energy."
Can you identify three problems you are having now? "Sleep cycle. So-
   cial interaction skills. That's it."

Can you identify three goals that you would like to accomplish while in the hospital? "To be able to make decisions with confidence and rapidity; engage in intellectual conversation. Feel good about myself."

Do you have any valuables for safekeeping? "Wristwatch, glasses."
Do you have any sharp objects with you? "Just my wit."
Do you have any medications with you? "No."
Habits: Denied alcohol or drug use. Does not smoke. No history of IVDA (intravenous drug use).

Do you have any sharp objects with you? "Just my wit."

I feel like Alice:

> "But I don't want to go among mad people," Alice remarked.
> "Oh, you can't help that," said the Cat: "We're all mad here. I'm mad, you're mad."
> "How do you know I'm mad?" said Alice.
> "You must be," said the Cat, "or you wouldn't have come here."
>
> —Lewis Carroll, *Alice's Adventures in Wonderland* (1865)

I am asked to disrobe and put on a piece of cloth known euphemistically as a hospital gown that leaves the back half of my anatomy exposed and frigid. After asking for two "gowns," I tie one in back and one in front, managing to cover all the body parts unaccustomed to public exposure. This has got to be some psychiatrist's idea of a joke, I mutter. They question a guy about gender identity and then hand him something called a gown.

As I move down the conveyer belt from one nurse to another, my clothing is itemized and bundled for transport to the hospital ward where I will eventually reside: "Jacket. T-shirt. Shirt. Underwear. Trousers. Shoes. Socks." I sign to verify that the itemized list is complete. Were my mind focusing on the here and now instead of the dull green walls of the ER, I might wonder whether my clothes were to be donated to Goodwill— a thought that should be of more concern to the guy who signed in (at almost the same time as I did) wearing the Armani jacket. But he and I now look like we've got the same tailor. And begowned, my chances of "escaping" my new guardians drop. "Doctor, how will we identify the escaped person who may be suffering from bipolar disorder?" "Well, officer, it should be pretty easy. Just look for someone who is barefoot and bare-assed running down the street wearing a white and green garment with a giant slit tied by a string in the back."

While waiting in an emergency reception area and then a padded room for four hours, I am subject to further scrutiny. I remember an ad jingle. "Sometimes you feel like a nut. Sometimes you don't." I don't feel like a nut. Where I had started the process feeling manic, I am now cycling back and forth. The molecules in my body seem to be spinning in a cyclotron one minute and shutting down the next. My Mental Status Examination:

> On admission, casually dressed male appearing stated age. Calm, cooperative with examination. Mood was sad. Affect was restricted. Positive psychomotor retardation. Speech was normal rate and tone. Thought process was disorganized and thought blocking was circumstantial. Denied any auditory or visual hallucinations. Denied any current suicidal ideation although admits to suicidal ideation two days prior to admission. Thought content was preoccupied with guilt about illness and burdening family. Judgment and insight poor.

An hour later a nurse writes: "Pt quite agitated banging hands and head on padded wall, a very testy affect." A resident, notepad and pencil in hand, asks me, "What is the year that we are in now? What is the date? What day is this? What month are we in? Count backward from 100 in units of 7. Spell *world* backward."

I am also asked for a urine and blood sample. Among other things, the men and women in white coats want to know my lithium level and whether I've been using illegal drugs that might interfere with my other medications or those that will be used in the hospital.

Amphetamines	Negative
Barbiturates	Negative
Benzodiazepines	Negative
COC Metabolite	Negative
Ethanol	Negative
Methadone	Negative
Opiates	Negative
PCP	Negative
THC	Negative
Lithium	.99

Those in the lab are also checking my blood and urine for signs of physical illness. My hematology (blood) profile is within normal range, as is my thyroid function. But the normal lithium level alarms me because that meant that lithium hadn't kept me well. After my earlier attempt to see whether I could remain illness free without lithium, I had taken it with almost religious fervor. In my mind, those pills stood between me and chaos. Now that assumption had been called into question.

In my mind, those pills stood between me and chaos. Now that assumption had been called into question.

I also sign a form that in effect surrenders some of my rights: "I give permission for performance of procedures that may be considered necessary or advisable for diagnosis and/or treatment of myself." Considered necessary by whom? Under what criteria? Perhaps this is a test to see whether the hospital can induce paranoia in someone suffering from bipolar disorder. I am too withdrawn to be offended by the second form either. It says that the hospital "may disclose any or all parts of the clinical record to my insurance company or employer for purposes of satisfying charges."

Between my first hospitalization and my last, federal confidentiality regulations (42 C.F.R. Part 2) were put in place that protect medical records containing psychiatric, drug abuse, or alcohol abuse treatment information. The form I signed in more recent admissions noted that

> The Federal rules prohibit the Hospital from making any further disclosure of this information/records unless further disclosure is expressly permitted by the patient's written consent or the consent of a person otherwise permitted by 42 C.F.R. Part 2. A general authorization for the release of medical or other information is NOT sufficient for this purpose. The Federal rules restrict any use of the information to criminally investigate or prosecute any alcohol or drug abuse patient.

I'm also asked to sign a form called "Consent for Voluntary Inpatient Treatment." By signing this form, I forfeit the right to leave the hospital against medical advice (AMA) without waiting a set period. During my six hospitalizations, the form asked for 72 hours notice before I could leave AMA. The form also stated that my rights as a patient have been described to me and that I consent to being treated. It's possible that someone has described my rights in agonizing detail, but if so I've lost any recollection of the experience in a manic wash or a depressive undertow.

As part of the ritual of being transformed from an independent citizen of the nonhospital world into a clearly identified patient, I am tagged like a bird with a wristband stating name and ID number. "You won't believe it, George," I imagine a bird watcher saying. "I saw a green-and-white-breasted manic depressive perched right over there in a wheelchair."

Finally, the paperwork is complete, the period of observation over, and someone has told someone else that the insurance company has agreed to cover the hospitalization. I am transported in a wheelchair to an "open" (unlocked) ward I will call "downstairs." The clothes I was wearing when I started this process four hours before bounce about in a sealed plastic bag on the back of the wheelchair as I'm wheeled to the elevator.

Twenty strangers locked in a house with one refrigerator, lousy food, a solitary confinement room with three-point restraints, and no phone (until you earn privileges). That's a psych ward. Twenty strangers who have in common a team of highly qualified professionals whose goal it is to get them well. That's a psych ward, too. At my hospital there was an open ward (downstairs) and a locked ward (upstairs).

A psychiatric ward consists of a door or series of doors monitored by someone who sits at command central—the nursing station. The open ward I was in had a small kitchen/dining area where patients ate breakfast, lunch, and dinner, a small exercise area with a stationary bicycle, a TV viewing area (the TV only had three channels), a small laundry area with a coin-operated washer and dryer, and a pool table. During one of my lengthy stays, the only beverage available was apple juice in tiny peel-off plastic containers. I didn't drink apple juice again for seven years. The large rectangular space that is the ward is ringed by patients' rooms. Psychiatric wards, like other wards except maternity, are coed.

During one of my lengthy stays, the only beverage available was apple juice . . . I didn't drink apple juice again for seven years.

The patients' rooms are small, spotless, functional, and subject to constant observation by the nursing staff. Mine has a single bed, a writing desk with a lamp, and a small nightstand. The room includes a washroom with sink and toilet. The window cannot be opened. A call button permits me to summon the nurse. There are no cords on the lamps and nothing in the room that could be fashioned into an instrument to be used to injure myself or someone else.

The person pushing the wheelchair into the ward hands my paperwork, the plastic bag of clothes, and me over to my primary nurse. I have reached the end of the conveyer belt. My name is entered on the large white board used to keep track of patient room assignments. As one shift leaves and another comes on duty, a record of my stay is passed along in written form:

> The patient was initially admitted to the unlock unit on the open ward and placed on special observations. The morning following admission the patient was noted to appear [with] increasingly unusual behavior. He began talking back at the overhead pager. I first met with the patient at this time. He appeared very disheveled, had minimal eye contact. Thoughts were fairly disorganized.

After walking with me to my room in the open ward at 4:00 A.M., my parents had gone home to get some sleep. What neither they nor I knew when I agreed to be admitted was that if in the judgment of those in charge I was a danger to myself or others on the open ward, I would be reassigned to the locked ward. Ditto if they should conclude that I planned to escape or, in the euphemism of the hospital, "elope":

> The patient began to express fears of being hurt or losing control of himself and potentially hurting someone else. After he gathered up all of his belongings from his room, he stood in the hallway, moving towards walking off the unit, the patient was asked if he would please return to his room, at which point, he somewhat violently threw his clothing on the floor. He was subsequently offered and agreed to medication. . . . He was subsequently transferred to the locked unit "upstairs" for potentially dangerous behavior as well as possible elopement risk.

Forcibly transferred to a locked ward, I felt betrayed.

The "Patient" Is a Risk . . .

If you are part of the non-hospitalized population, you seek entrance to the locked ward "upstairs" by identifying yourself on an intercom outside a first door. A voice acknowledges you and tells you that you can come in. A buzzer indicates that the lock on the first door has been opened. You walk through, head down a hallway, and confront a second door. On the other side of that door is the world of the hypervigilant. Once you are in, you can only leave if someone at the nursing station "buzzes you through." Those from the outside world who are not being admitted as patients must check in at the nurses' station. If they are bearing gifts for a patient, those items are checked and either approved or held. Trojan horses are not welcome. The non-hospitalized population also stops at the nurses' station before leaving. If you are part of either the hospitalized or non-hospitalized population and need some attention, simply bolt for the door. In a psychiatric hospital, running will get you noticed, no matter who you are.

In a psychiatric hospital, running will get you noticed, no matter who you are.

My mother found out that I had been transferred when she showed up for visiting hours the next afternoon and instead of locating me on the open ward was directed to the locked ward. Drugged into a deep sleep, I didn't know she was there.

> Mother and father [express] discomfort with son being on a locked ward with "bizarre people." . . . Parents express anger, frustration and feelings of abandonment by medical staff/system.

I emerge from my drugged stupor into a world unlike one I have ever imagined. In a locked ward, patients' rights are severely restricted; the atmosphere is less than friendly. Locked wards have a physical restraint room and an isolation (or "seclusion") room, places where you end up if you don't follow directions or you break floor rules (e.g., touching another patient). And they're scary places—so much so that I've decided those who call the padded isolation room a "seclusion" room, as if it were a zenlike mountain retreat, suffer from an impairment that, if I were to write my own version of the *DSM* (the *DSM-PJ*), would be called "compulsive euphemization." Solitary confinement, perhaps, but seclusion!?

It is freaky being surrounded by disoriented strangers. I get a jumbled feeling in my stomach when I listen to other patients' despair about how much pain they are in and how their doctors are lying to them. Some don't have visitors. Others are unaware of the visitors they do have. There is a continuum in terms of the quality of my psychiatric nursing care. For some nurses, it is their calling, while others are burned out and much less pleasant to deal with.

> The mind is its own place, and in itself can make a Heaven of Hell, a Hell of Heaven.
>
> —John Milton, *Paradise Lost* (1667)

On this locked ward, an authoritarian alpha male nurse with a handle bar mustache named Jack delights in beating the heavily sedated patients at chess. Even though my departing gift from the open ward nurses, an overly large injection of the antipsychotic Haldol, makes my joints stiff and is still clouding my mind, I delude myself into thinking that by winning this game I can beat my illness, escape my jailer, and win my freedom. I feel like Sisyphus pushing the boulder uphill, my hands slipping with each loss of my pawns, knights, and rook, until my black queen falls and the boulder rolls back over my mind. I feel alone, in ruins, and my hope for release that day dies.

Each morning as part of "morning rounds," a group of medical students guided by a doctor appears in my room. I have become a visual aid in a teaching process: "Pt. expressed discomfort about forum of morning rounds and being 'stared at by a group of would-be doctors (residents).'" In the 1970s doctors in this same ward actually spent quality time working with the patients. Twenty years later these visits had been knocked down to about 30 seconds.

Psychiatrists see the world through the lens of psychiatry. The residents refer to me as the bipolar in 302. One doctor asked, "How are we feeling today?" "Aha!" I thought. "A test to see whether I think I am two different people." When I responded, "I'm feeling tired but have no idea how you are feeling," he seemed annoyed.

Because hospitals are noisy places, getting to sleep can be complicated. During one hospitalization, my neighbor's snoring, which sounded like a baby crying, kept me awake. Another time, a neighboring patient dry heaved into his toilet until early in the morning. I used earplugs to block out the sounds of the hospital when they were keeping me awake at night. During the day, when I couldn't focus well enough to read, I listened to music.

Encounters with hostile patients are frightening. I've been threatened, had food thrown at me, and observed a patient I'll call Johnny chew off part of his own lip, and get tackled, drugged, and put in restraints for three days. Freed from the restraints, Johnny responded to his confinement and further endeared himself to the ward by urinating at the crack under the door, flooding the hallway we walked through. Another time, a middle-aged female patient told me in a conspiratorial tone that we were all about to be transported off the planet by a spaceship that would land on the roof of the hospital. Had that occurred, it certainly would have enlivened my hospital stay. Then again, for part of my time in the locked ward, I was so out of it that it's possible I was whisked to another planet and back and never knew the difference.

In the course of the move to the locked ward "upstairs," I was placed on special observation, a category that means my location and activities were checked in 15-minute intervals. During one four-hour period, my "psychiatric nursing special observation flow sheet" reports that I spent from 0015-0100 asleep in my room, from 0115-0130 in my room awake, from 0145-0245 asleep in my room. At 0300 I was in the hall, at 0315 in my room awake, and from 0315-0415 asleep again. Seeing my life charted in units of 15 minutes, which I was able to do when I secured release of my medical records, was among the stranger experiences involved in gathering the material for this book. The strangest was realizing how inexact the process of translating my life onto the paper of the medical records is. My psychiatrist's name is spelled five different ways; he is confused with my primary care physician; and, in what I assume was a typing error, one hospital record indicates next to race that I am black (I'm white).

One of the rules of the psych ward is that a patient requires permission to engage in activities that in the outside world are taken for granted. Since the staff is fearful that I could try to hang myself, I must request a shower hose and secure permission to take a shower. Because I am under special observation, a nurse keeps an eye on me while I

One of the rules of the psych ward is that a patient requires permission to engage in activities that in the outside world are taken for granted.

shower. Rules depend on who is enforcing them and on that particular day the only personal items permitted in my room are a toothbrush, toothpaste, and comb. Disposable razors are contraband. Shaving requires permission. When you are not under special observation you are allowed to have more personal items.

The process of "getting well" entails an increasing level of responsibility that takes the form of "privileges." Being permitted to change out of a hospital gown into street clothes is a privilege. Not wanting a scruffy hospital beard, I must ask permission to shave.

During one of my hospitalizations, I was asked to participate in a study. In the proposed study, I would forego sleep for a night. The literature says relief of depression by interrupting R.E.M. sleep is short-lived and exhausts the patient. Theoretically, medications should be able to stabilize this new depression-less state, but I have never heard of lithium or any other mood-elevating drug acting in less than ten days. I am very suspicious of hospital studies. When in doubt I stay away from them no matter how much I want to please my doctor, nurse, or resident. The open-ended permission that I signed to be admitted didn't cover experiments. It only covers procedures that are medically necessary. Hence, "when told he would need to stay up tonight for a sleep deprived EEG, he refused adamantly and his mother states, 'I don't want that for him.'" Those who wanted my cooperation in the study backed off when I refused.

Because I am writing this while neither manic nor depressed, I may be failing to convey the reasons I was admitted to the hospital in the first place. There are times when your sense that you are well should be subjected to impartial confirmation by others around you. Once when hospitalized, I informed a doctor that I thought I was ready to go home. Deadpan, she responded, "Perhaps we should wait for a day in which you did not take a shower with your clothes on." She laughed when I recommended *One Flew Over the Cuckoo's Nest* as our weekly movie. "There's such high demand for it," she commented. "It's probably checked out."

Sailing the Bureaucracy of Boredom

You're only given a little spark of madness. You mustn't lose it.

—Attributed to Robin Williams

Why did I "act out" a few times while hospitalized? Picture yourself on a seemingly never-ending voyage that costs two to three thousand dollars a day. Your craft is the U.S.S. *Monotony*, the flagship of the insomnia class of submarines. Because of her 15-minute bed checks, she is designed to ensure that you are unable to sleep without meds that make you feel even worse. She serves unlimited apple juice in tiny containers, or tap water if you can find a cup, and there are only three TV channels in the meeting area—including one that shows *The People's Court,* reminding you that back on land it is a good idea to sue your neighbor for $1.49 because his goose ate your flowers. All your neighbors are drugged up, and no one will talk to you long enough to have a meaningful conversation, especially the staff, who have other things to do. After several weeks of this, during one of my hospital stays, some would say I decided to liven this voyage up a bit, while others would note that I lost control for a few minutes.

I decided that it would be rip-roaring funny if I put my underwear on my head and jogged around the psych ward as if I were crazy.

After protesting that I no longer needed to be hospitalized, my behavior confirmed that the outside world was not yet ready for my sense of reality. I decided that it would be rip-roaring funny if I put my underwear on my head and jogged around the psych ward as if I were crazy. By my logic at the time, if I could distinguish between being crazy and acting crazy, I'd feel better. By demonstrating that I was only pretending to be crazy, the stigma associated with hospitalization (and supposedly being crazy) would be wiped clean.

Where I saw myself as a happy-go-lucky guy protesting the insanity and utter boredom of the psych ward, the nurse in charge saw my behavior not as an indication of ironic commentary, but as a sign of psychosis. In that case, her reality was probably closer to that of the rest of the world than mine. I was given the choice of "the pill" (a large dose of antipsychotic) or some unspecified consequence. I chose the pill. Previously, I had been pinned down and shoved (with a syringe) for lesser infractions than wearing a new kind of headgear. If I had refused the pill, they would have pinned me, shoved the needle in, and juiced me on Haldol.

Sometimes in the hospital the word *psychotic* was deployed with a visceral ease that I resented. A few residents who visited me mistook my practicing French verb conjugations for a class as meaning I was psychotic. (When in a psych ward, those in charge often talk about you as if you are not there. I would add this to my own version of the *DSM*, the *DSM-PJ*, as "disappearance syndrome." Where other psychotics see things that aren't there, those with this syndrome don't see things that are.)

I have had some French teachers who were eccentric, but I never interpreted their tendency to move in and out of the language as a forecast of mental collapse. *Mais, non!*

Is Getting Weirder Normal?

With the level of strange behavior in psych wards, I'm surprised that those employed there haven't developed a broader sense of the so-called "normal." There are exceptions. One nurse, for example, observed, "Pt continues disorganized speech peppered with puns and jokes and random philosophical observations. 'If you are altruistic that contradicts Darwinism.'" Another observed:

> Speaks with occasional evidence of perplexity, severe distractibility, but episodes of acutely observed, witty commentary or response, essentially one liners delivered with moderate pressure of speech and heightened sense of hilarity. However he was able to attend sufficiently to complete tomorrow's menu, and give me minimal assessment data. In the latter, masked hostility was evident in content at time but overt behavior was playful.

As loathe as I am to write the sentence, one advantage that I had upon returning to the ward in which I had stayed in the past was that the staff had some experience with me when I was closer to well. That provides an interpretive context that is useful in distinguishing so-called "abnormal," and hence worrisome, verbal behavior from so-called "normal" verbal statements—the sort I make routinely when fully functional in the non-hospital world.

One of the problems with being hospitalized is that those in charge require you to confirm you're sick as a sign that you are getting well. Arguing that you are well enough to go home can

. . . those in charge require you to confirm you're sick as a sign that you are getting well.

as a result be interpreted as a sign that you're not ready at all. Indeed, insisting that you are now able to function adequately outside the confines of the hospital can be taken as a signal that you are in denial about your illness. As my records indicate:

> The family dynamics seem to be the greatest problem at this time. Parents and son do not acknowledge risk he presents to himself if he follows impulse to elope. Patient shows poor judgment and insight into severity of his illness as do parents at this time. "He might as well be at home."

How does one establish that one is getting well? A few days later, a nurse writes, "Pt does not realize or want to confront how sick he was on admission. Judgment: Pt currently agreeing to stay in hosp. Shows better judgment in interview setting."

How does one get transferred back to the open ward? The doctor in charge writes, "I do not believe him to be suicidal or elopement risk . . . transfer to the open ward."

Once back on the open ward, I have to deal with the same people who sent me away my first night there. Those on the open ward begin the process of persuading me that I am welcome on the open ward and was sent to the locked ward for what they saw as good reasons: "Pt does not appear to remember that . . . his open ward R.N. spoke to him extensively on the day of transfer about the reasons for transfer." Now in addition to figuring out why I hadn't managed the disorder well enough to remain unhospitalized, I am also trying to make sense of a process that seems to have done me in: "Pt appears focused on the negative aspects of his hospitalization, i.e., being drugged [and] taken upstairs."

However, by comparison to Johnny the "problem patient," I was an altar boy. When he wasn't peeing at the crack between the door and floor of the isolation room in order to dissolve the floor and escape, he was throwing food at the walls. I don't know what was going on in the world he was experiencing but suspect that he either thought he was Houdini or Jackson Pollock. The nurses on the ward concluded, and probably rightly so, that he was psychotic. Why put someone with that diagnosis in isolation? Perhaps some day someone with more degrees than I will explain that one to me. From my perspective, since their treatments for him were ineffective, I saw the doctors and nurses putting him in the "seclusion room" as a way of making their lives easier. If I didn't know Johnny better, I'd say he shared my sense of humor.

Part of my time in the hospital was spent readjusting medications. Part was spent learning about the disorder and how to cope with it: "Pt counseled about suicide risk with bipolar disorder as people start to have more energy." Part was spent in occupational therapy. When asked my goal in occupational therapy, I reported, "I want to be able to have a conversation." Part was spent in art therapy. One art therapy class during my last hospitalization in the 1990s was my first exposure to tai chi, a series of controlled dance-like moves including "fighting the monkey." In another, I sanded a piece of wood to fashion a stool. In a third, we cut colored paper into patterns with safety scissors.

Time moves slowly when you have nothing to do, when you are having a conversation with a boring boor, and when you are hospitalized. In the first two circumstances, I leave my watch on but glance at it repeatedly. In the last, I give my watch to a close friend or family member. That move prevents me from constantly checking the time. The ritual ends when I am discharged and put my watch back on.

Just as there was paperwork involved in being admitted, there is paperwork involved in being discharged. My patient discharge form includes instructions: "Take your medications as prescribed by your M.D. Maintain your outpatient therapy. Call your doctor if you experience a loss of energy, motivation, disorganization, thoughts of suicide, extended periods of sad or low mood." It also certifies that my "valuables" (like my wallet) and belongings (like my clothing) have been returned to me. Finally, it records my temperature, pulse, respiration, and blood pressure—an assurance that on departure I was physically healthy.

I look at my hospitalizations as follows. I had the "choice" of getting even sicker or checking into the hospital and getting better. I was very fortunate to have this option, and like many other patients my condition improved during each hospitalization. Though I am thankful for the opportunity to heal, after being discharged six times, I vowed that I would do everything I could to ensure that I would not need to be readmitted. Ever.

> *I look at my hospitalizations as follows. I had the "choice" of getting even sicker or checking into the hospital and getting better.*

Stigma

There is a stigma associated with a diagnosis of mental disorder, an additional stigma attached to seeing a psychiatrist, and an even greater stigma associated with hospitalization for a mental disorder. In one 1992 survey by the National Mental Health Association (NMHA), nearly half of the public reported that it sees depression not as an illness but a defect in character! Among those who stigmatized mental illness were some who reported that they were more likely than average to have felt depressed at least monthly. A NMHA poll conducted in 1996 found that more than half (54%) "believe that depression is a sign of weakness, not an illness."

Beliefs of this sort, beliefs that assign shame to an illness, are partly what stigma is about. They're based in ignorance and fear and can do irreparable harm by preventing those with a serious mental illness from getting help (including hospitalization) because doing so might mark them as "crazy" or "weak" or "defective" or whatever adjective people use to distance themselves from those they don't understand. One goal for this book is to debunk myths about mental illness—and bipolar disorder in particular—to reduce the stigma associated with it, and by openly describing my experiences, to encourage others with the illness to seek help. There is evidence that suggests that believing you can get well makes it more likely you will get help—in spite of stigma and discrimination against the mentally ill. It is important to remember that hospitalization and other therapies can be a necessary and healing element in your life. Simply put, don't allow small-minded stigma and prejudice to prevent you from taking advantage of these therapeutic options if you and your doctors deem it necessary.

Once out of the hospital, I confront questions about my absence and preconceptions of where I was. It's tempting to say "none of your business" when acquaintances ask where you've been. Or to report "on a Caribbean cruise." If it is none of their business, I usually reply, "I just needed some peace and quiet."

It hurts when people say I've been in the "nuthouse" or "funny farm" instead of the hospital. I realize that they mean to be funny, but there's nothing funny about the funny farm.

I think it is important, especially if you are young and have a mental disorder, to establish or join a responsible peer group so you can reflect, vent, and plan actions to deal with the hostility the world throws at those of us who are different (see the Resources section for information on peer support groups). Bullies often pick on people who are isolated, and one of the common traits of happy people is that they are social. So if you force yourself to be social, even if you are low energy, you have a better shot at feeling better. Plan activities and stay social!

I am lucky because I have health insurance and access to outpatient mental health care. Unfortunately, America uses its jail system instead of hospitals to treat many poor and mentally ill people. In July 1999, newspapers around the country reported that "[t]he first comprehensive study of the rapidly growing number of emotionally disturbed people in the nation's jails and prisons . . . found that there are 283,800 inmates with mental illness, about 16 percent of the jail population." An article in the *New York Times* noted in 1999, "The report confirms the belief of many state, local and Federal experts that jails and prisons have become the nation's new mental hospitals." According to the study, conducted by the Justice Department, "mentally ill inmates tend to follow a revolving door from *homelessness* to incarceration and then back to the streets with little treatment, many of them arrested for crimes that grow out of their illnesses." Where there were 559,000 individuals in state hospitals in 1955, 40 years later there were 69,000. We need to commit the resources to make a national health plan that properly addresses mental health a reality.

The point is that hospitalization should be readily available to everyone who needs it, and that need shouldn't be sloughed off as a joke. Before anyone uses the terms "loony bin" or "funny farm," they should visit a psychiatric ward. They'll find people who are disoriented, depressed, and confused, suffering from mania, but mostly just medicated and working on getting their medical illness under control so they can return to their lives. Under those circumstances, we are bored, frightened, and often lonely. Most of all we are ill. There is nothing "crazy" about asking for help when ill. Keep repeating: I need lithium just as someone with diabetes needs insulin; and at this moment I need the intensive treatment from the hospital environment. Unfortunately there's a stigma associated with both. But the stigma says more about the ignorance of those who hold it than it says about us or our condition.

There is nothing "crazy" about asking for help when ill.

Chapter Six

The Illness Is Not Our Identity

I feel like I'm taking CRAZY PILLS!

—Will Ferrell playing Mugatu in *Zoolander* (2001)

Our disorder falls into a widely misunderstood category of illnesses. This chapter could be titled, "What Should I Call It? What Should I Call Myself?" I believe we should take command of the language because words help frame the way we see the world. And people see us in part through the labels we apply and those applied to us.

Words, Words, and More Words:
The Tyranny of Labels

First, let's take on name-calling. We are not loonies or looney tunes, fruitloops, fruitcakes, or nut cases. Although I occasionally bay at a full moon (or *luna* in Latin) and regard with suspicion those who don't, I'm not a lunatic either. We aren't nuts or screwy. Nor do I have a screw loose (a few bolts and cotter pins perhaps, but no screws). Screwballs are found in ballparks, not psychiatric wards. We are *mental,* but so is everyone who functions cognitively. We are not crazy or crazed. By the way, you can refer to your bipolar disorder as a "chemical imbalance" if you think people in your school, work, or family will be less likely to say hurtful things.

When I was 16, I resented the term "high" as a description of my manic state. It sounded as if I were doing drugs even though I had smoked about as much dope as Bill Clinton (except I did inhale). It also implied that being in a manic state was illegal or immoral.

Thankfully, *maniac* is no longer the noun of preference when referring to those experiencing mania. Not too long ago, it was. In 1930, psychoanalyst Karl Menninger concluded a discussion of a patient by writing, "The extreme of the 'up phase' is called *mania*; Jane was, technically, a maniac."

In psychiatry, *mania* is a word of much splendor. Its possible prefixes signal a range of behaviors. You've probably heard of egomania (being preoccupied with oneself) and kleptomania (coveting thy neighbor's goods in the extreme), but you may be less familiar with trichotillomania—compulsively yanking out one's hair.

The mania of bipolar disorder falls in the category of affective or mood disorders. Say that you have an "affective disorder" and most will hear the statement as an oxymoron—a contradiction: "effective disorder." Better, I suppose, than an ineffective one. "Mood disorder" suggests that you are cranky or not in the mood.

I have a problem with the terms used to describe this illness or disorder. For example, just because the condition is called bipolar disorder or manic depression doesn't mean that we are manic depressives, disordered, or bipolar. The earth is bipolar. I am not. A polar bear attracted to both the

. . . just because the condition is called bipolar disorder or manic depression doesn't mean that we are manic depressives, disordered, or bipolar.

male and the female of his species is bipolar. I am not (bipolar or attracted to both the male and female of my species). My bedroom is disorderly; I am neither disorderly nor disordered. *The condition is not my identity.* It is an adjective, not a noun, in my life. Note the difference between the following sentences:

> I have brown eyes and hair, asthma, and flat feet, and I am near-sighted and experience occasional manic and depressive episodes.
>
> I am a manic depressive with brown eyes and hair who is near-sighted, asthmatic, and has flat feet.

In the second sentence, the condition is *the* defining element in my life. In the first, the condition is instead a descriptive fact, which is no more central to my identity than many others.

Unless I have laser surgery, I will wear glasses or contacts for the rest of my life. I will take lithium for the rest of my life unless the equivalent of laser surgery is discovered for bipolar disorder. But I am not the illness and the illness is not me.

If you must think of me in terms of an illness, please call me a person with a bipolar condition, and emphasize *person*. I have thousands of characteristics that taken together define me, and this condition is only one of them. It's not, in other words, some alien presence that takes me over and remakes me, an invasion of the mind snatcher. It is not a replacement or a substitute for me.

I want to be an agent rather than a patient. A patient is passive by definition. Unless I am in the hospital, I prefer that therapists think of me as a client because it stresses my autonomy and the extent to which I can exert control in the treatment process. I'm not alone in rejecting the phrase *mental patient*, a passive label, in favor of such active terms as *consumer* and *client*.

Some who do use the term *patient* express discomfort about it. For instance, psychotherapist T. B. Karasu wrote in 1992, "I often still use the unfortunate word *patient*. I would like to redefine the concept to broaden its connotations, or, failing that, at least to neutralize the term. My hope is that the word will be spared the stigmatic or social status associations that define the therapist-patient relationship."

The word *client* also is a reminder that psychiatry is a service I purchase, either directly or through health insurance. Additionally, it reminds me that I have choices in the doctors or therapists I select and the treatments I adopt. Another term freighted with submission is *compliance*. That term typically refers to the extent to which patients, as one psychology reference book put it in 1998, "obediently and faithfully follow health care providers' instructions, assignments, and prescriptions. By contrast, the term *adherence* implies a more active, voluntary, and collaborative involvement of the patient in a mutually acceptable course of behavior that produces a desired preventive or therapeutic result." Amen.

One of the problems in talking about bipolar disorder is that its names have been adopted by the culture to describe normal swings in emotion. I feel fine today. There are days (and nights) when I feel "down" or "up," but neither state would be appropriately described as a pole that is part of the label *bipolar* or as *depression* or *mania*. Just because I'm tired and quiet at the end of a long day doesn't mean that I'm DEPRESSED. Just because I'm particularly excited, creative, and spontaneous doesn't mean that I'm MANIC. But in a world filled with people who know little about this condition, the words *depressed* and *manic* are used all the time and meant in the lowercase sense. "I'm really depressed about the grade I got on that test," says a student. "The kids were really manic today," says a teacher.

While we're on the subject of language, let's not ignore the verbs. I'm not, for example, particularly fond of the notion that "I suffer from bipolar illness or manic depression." I am not a martyr. Nor do I welcome the notion that "I am afflicted by the illness." It is not, after all, the plague.

"Suffer" and "afflicted by" also cast me as the object on which the disease acts as if it were a superhuman alien and I a pliant victim. Don't get me wrong. I'm not telling you that I welcome this condition or that I'd cling to it if I had the option to jettison it. But facts are facts. And the fact is that this condition and I sometimes inhabit the same space. But our relationship is not a defining one. Instead of saying "I am," or "I have," I prefer "I feel": "I feel manic," or "I feel depressed." Most of the time, I feel fine.

But not all of the time. At least not all of the time in the same way. *Chronic* is an odd word and in some ways inadequate to describe this condition. In a world that divides medical conditions into the well and the ill, are we well when not manic or depressed? Or are we ill? I'd rather reserve "ill" for times in which I feel manic or depressed and say the rest of the time that I have the condition but not the illness. Why should I conclude that I have an "illness" when on most days of most months of most years I feel fine—and can't be picked out of a crowd even by a psychiatrist trained to spot cues signaling the condition? If you want to use the word *illness* (e.g., "I have manic-depressive illness"), why not reserve it for the times that you feel and act ill? In fact, I'm drawn to the phrases "manic episode" and "depressive episode" because "episode" brackets the illness, suggesting that it is a transitory, impermanent state, and invites others to think of the condition as something other than my identity.

> I'd rather reserve "ill" for times in which I feel manic or depressed and say the rest of the time that I have the condition but not the illness.

So what do I say about my condition? The answer is "as little as possible to as few as possible," because it is as much somebody else's business as the fact that I am nearsighted. But when the need to describe the condition arises, my preference is to say, "I take lithium to minimize the effects of a chemical imbalance in the brain known as manic depression or bipolar disorder."

As the person with the condition, I have the right to determine what I will call it. My description and yours may vary. For example, Dr. Kay Redfield Jamison, coauthor of a definitive medical text called *Manic-Depressive Illness* and a person who also has the condition, said that she prefers "manic-depressive" to "bipolar" because it better characterizes the mixed states and extremes of the illness.

Whatever it's called, the condition isn't in charge of me. To the extent possible, I am in charge of it. Instead of a label describing the states that one can experience (manic depression), I prefer a description of what is going on (chemical imbalance being treated by lithium). Those with diabetes take insulin to correct an imbalance in their secretion of insulin; I take lithium to correct an imbalance in the chemicals in my brain.

Additionally, some talk about bipolar disorder as if it belongs to them. They do so with such phrases as "my illness" and "I have bipolar disorder." These phrases seem strange to me. My cat, my hat, my illness? I have a cat and a hat, but I do not have bipolar disorder. The illness is not mine—it is shared by up to 1% of Americans. It is in my brain. It is an "illness" when I'm ill with it; it is a "condition" when I'm not.

How can one describe the experience of mania or depression? Author, war veteran, and a person who has battled depression, William Styron commented in his book *Darkness Visible* that the language we use to describe horrible pain and suffering is inappropriate when it comes to depression and manic depression. We need a term that communicates some of what we go through with this condition. *Melancholia* is anachronistic, literally meaning black bile; *depression* isn't right either. It's too pretty a word.

We need more evocative words than *depression* and *mania* to express the illness. Surely a versatile language such as English houses a better term, perhaps one with hard consonants. I suggest *wracknation*. For example, "James experienced a week of wracknation before he could brush his teeth and shower unassisted." Styron had the same kind of impulse, calling depression "a true wimp of a word for such a major illness."

Language does evolve. There have been important alterations in the ways the world talks about us and our condition. "'Possession' (demoniac) became 'bewitchery,'" wrote Menninger in 1963, then "'bewitchery' became 'madness,' 'madness' became 'lunacy,' 'lunacy' became 'insanity,' 'insanity' became 'psychosis,' a word many of us feel to be no more scientific than the word 'bewitched.'"

Some have theorized that the harshness of the diagnosis is inversely correlated with the thickness of one's wallet. For example, in 1932 French psychiatrist Pierre Janet noted that the poor who were sent to the public mental hospital were called "psychotic," while those who could afford care in a private sanatorium were said to suffer "neurasthenia," and those sufficiently wealthy to be treated at home were said to be indisposed and called "eccentric"

Just as *drunk* has given way to *alcoholic*, words such as *crazy, lunatic,* and *insane* have given way to others with clinical definitions. *Depression* is different, for example, from *manic depression.* Society has also abandoned some of the language used to connote

Just as drunk has given way to alcoholic, words such as crazy, lunatic, and insane have given way to others with clinical definitions.

the horrors of past treatments of those with mental illness. These changes in language reflect changes in treatment. Instead of insane asylums and mental institutions, we now have psychiatric wards and hospitals.

The Self-Fulfilling Prophecy and Misconceptions About Violence

Names and labels matter. Each time I have signed into a psychiatric ward, my identity became that of someone with bipolar illness, and "someone with bipolar illness" became a defining part of who I was to others. Outside the hospital, I could feature my identity as a husband, father, brother, son, student, scuba diver, horseback rider, researcher, and author. Once inside, doctors and nurses identified me only by my diagnosis, and treated me accordingly. The danger is that both in and outside the hospital, the stereotypes about mental illness become the reality in what is known as a self-fulfilling prophecy. Others construct a set of assumptions based on stereotypes about mental illness, and eventually we become the stereotype because it is human nature to do or be what is "expected."

The notion of self-fulfilling prophecy was identified by Columbia University sociologist Robert Merton in an essay published in 1948. A self-fulfilling prophecy occurs "when an originally false social belief leads to its own fulfillment . . . [W]hen a self-fulfilling prophecy occurs, perceivers' initially erroneous social beliefs cause targets to act in ways that *objectively* confirm those beliefs."

In a 1968 experiment testing the power of self-fulfilling prophecies, researchers told teachers that some of their elementary school students were "late bloomers" whose performance and test scores would improve dramatically as the year progressed. In fact, the students given this designation by the researchers had been randomly selected. There was no reason to believe that their performance would differ from the others in the class. In a finding they called the Pygmalion effect, the IQs of the students who were labeled "late bloomers" did in fact increase.

The study raised questions about the extent to which social beliefs affect social reality. If the social beliefs are persistent and reinforced by the wider culture, their effect is likely to be greater than it would be otherwise. Media portrayals like those in Hitchcock's movie *Psycho,* for example, in which the killer Norman Bates is called mentally ill, reinforce stereotypes about violence and the mentally ill. Unfortunately, it's a stereotype that lingers even in the minds of the very young: According to the National Annenberg Risk Survey of Youth conducted in 2002, more than 65% of polled Americans between the ages of 14 and 22 reported believing that those with bipolar disorder are more likely to be violent than those without the disorder, and more than 55% reported believing in this likelihood among those with depression as well. One possible explanation for this common perception that a psychiatric patient will prove violent could be the pervasive use of the mentally ill criminal as a plot device in books and movies, and the inclusion of a psychiatric diagnosis in accounts of those who killed themselves.

But in fact, despite what we see when we read a news headline or watch a movie, mentally ill people are not necessarily violent. In an issue of *Psychiatric News* from May 2001, Dr. Otto Wahl wrote, "mental illness is a poor predictor of violence, ranking well after these factors: youth, male gender, history of violence, or poverty. Aside from people who abuse substances, people with mental illness commit violent acts at the same rate as non-patients, and 80 percent to 90 percent of people with mental illness never commit violent acts."

Stigma Revisited

Even those who are highly educated can perpetuate stereotypes about mental illness. *A Brotherhood of Tyrants*, written in 1994, claims that, "What drove them all [Hitler, Napoleon, and Stalin] to power, enabled them to gain it, and then carried them beyond reason was precisely the same disorder—manic depression— which in all three cases manifested itself in startlingly similar ways. Hitler, Napoleon, and Stalin's rise to power and subse- quent behavior was driven by their manic depression." How does it feel to be lumped in the same category as Hitler and Stalin?

Statements stigmatizing mental illness produce scorn instead of support for those with the illness. History's greatest villains did not attain power because of their manic depression. The condition is or may have been one of their characteristics, not their identity. It is appalling to suggest that millions might have been saved if only Hitler, Napoleon, and Stalin had been treated. *A Brotherhood of Tyrants* ignores their determination, intellect, and the historical happenstance of their being in the right place (one might say the wrong place) at the right time. *Brotherhood* also underplays the disabling effects of a condition that includes debilitating depressions. Labeling three of history's most noto- rious dictators as manic depressives says that the condition de- fined who they were and, as such, explains their actions.

If someone wants to argue that some of history's monsters had bipolar disorder, it's important to respond that some of history's geniuses had depression or bipolar disorder. As Aristotle noted in the fourth century B.C., "Those who have become eminent in philosophy, [politics, poetry, and the arts] have all had tendencies toward melancholia." Sir Isaac Newton, Rob- ert Lowell, Ernest Hemingway, Jack London, Abraham Lin- coln, Sylvia Plath, and, for the macho set, George Patton, had

Sir Isaac Newton, Robert Lowell, Ernest Hemingway, Jack London, Abraham Lincoln, Sylvia Plath, and, for the macho set, George Patton, had some of the problems we face.

some of the problems we face. Despite the fact that most of them didn't have lithium and antidepressants, they led incredible lives. So can we. We remember Newton for gravity, Lowell for "Colloquy in Black Rock," Hemingway for *The Old Man and the Sea*, London for *The Call of the Wild*, Lincoln for leading the country through the Civil War, Plath for her visceral and brilliant poetry, and Patton for his leadership during World War II.

None of them were defined by this condition. We shouldn't be either. Three of their lives ended in suicide. From that we should take a warning. This condition can be powerful. But so can we.

Chapter Seven

One in Two Million

All my growth and development led me to believe that if you really
do the right thing, and if you play by the rules, and if you've got
good enough, solid judgment and common sense, that you're going
to be able to do whatever you want to do with your life.

—the Hon. Barbara Jordan, former member
of the U.S House of Representatives

If you're 14 to 19 and angry, been there, done that. If you've
been misdiagnosed and nearly killed by a reaction to a prescribed drug, been there and done that, too. I've also suffered
embarrassing social situations because I couldn't stop talking
or was too depressed to say anything at all. And, yes, I know
about the relationships that shatter when someone can't handle
being the friend of someone with a chronic illness. It's neither
fair nor our fault. We can respond by sulking or by making the
best of it. In an attempt to make the best of it, we're in some
pretty distinguished company. In the last chapter I mentioned
just a few of the people in history who, given contemporary
diagnostic labels, could have been diagnosed with bipolar disorder yet who led accomplished, full lives that benefited the
world in some meaningful way. In this chapter, let me mention
just a few people with the illness who are making notable con-
tributions of their own today.

Three Distinguished People Who Have Bipolar Disorder

I'm not related to Dr. Kay Redfield Jamison, the expert on manic depression. My last name is an "e" away from hers. I first learned of Jamison by reading her classic text, *Manic-Depressive Illness* (1990), which she wrote with Dr. Frederick Goodwin, and then by finding her book *Touched with Fire* (1993), which shows that the illness is linked to creativity. In April 1995, Jamison acknowledged in an interview with the *Washington Post* that she has manic-depressive illness. "To some," wrote neuropsychiatrist Nancy Andreasen in 1995 in the *Washington Post*, "her disclosure would be a shock; to others, it would be nothing more than a confirmed assumption. But it was likely to be a big deal in psychiatric circles, where the fear of being perceived as crazier than one's patients is very real and very stigmatizing, and clinical privileges can be jeopardized for political rather than medical reasons." Jamison, who had first experienced the disorder at 16, is a professor at Johns Hopkins University. When she spoke at the Free Library (the main public library in Center City, Philadelphia) in 1997, the place was packed. From my seat in the back of the auditorium, I reminded myself, "She's been through it, too. She's made it. I can, too."

From my seat in the back of the auditorium, I reminded myself, "She's been through it, too. She's made it. I can, too."

In 1976, Ted Turner purchased the Atlanta Braves. In 1977, he skippered the sailboat that won the America's Cup. He is a person of multiple accomplishments. Among other things, he changed the face of television by realizing that he could use a satellite positioned in permanent orbit to send signals to the world 24 hours a day. CNN is no longer derided as the "Chicken Noodle Network."

A person of vision and high energy, Turner also has a reputation for cutting his opponents no slack. Porter Bibb's book *It Ain't as Easy as It Looks* describes a 1983 magazine interview in which Turner, when asked about his claim that "CBS is a cheap whorehouse run by sleaze artists," explained, "I'm up some days and down others. Some days, I just refuse comment. If I'm feeling a little down, I won't say anything. But if I'm really up, I'll let it all hang out. I do have a slight propensity to put my foot in my mouth."

Although he did not know it at the time, you and I can see mania written all over Turner's comments. Two years later, he was diagnosed with bipolar disorder and began seeing a therapist and taking lithium. A friend later described the change in Turner in a 1992 article in *Time* magazine: "Before, it was pretty scary to be around the guy sometimes because you never knew what in the world was going to happen next. If he was about to fly off the handle, you just never knew. That's why the whole world was on pins and needles around him . . . But with lithium he became very even tempered. Ted's just one of those miracle cases. I mean, lithium is great stuff, but in Ted's particular case, lithium is a miracle." In 1992, *Time* named Turner "Man of the Year."

"If resumes were automobiles," wrote reporter Laurel Shackelford, Bob Boorstin's "would be a Rolls-Royce. A Harvard graduate who polished off his education at Cambridge University in England, he easily landed a reporting job at the *New York Times* soon after graduation." At age 27, Boorstin was diagnosed with bipolar disorder. He was hospitalized for it once in 1987 and once the year after. When he went to a hospital the second time at the recommendation of his psychiatrist, Boorstin was told that he had exceeded the lifetime limit on his health insurance for the treatment of mental health. "Eventually someone reached Boorstin's brother on Wall Street, and using his American Express Card, he provided the $18,000 the hospital demanded." Boorstin filed suit against the hospital for denying coverage. He won and gained coverage equal to that allowed for so-called physical illnesses.

He then worked for Democratic presidential nominee Michael Dukakis in 1988 and Bill Clinton in 1992. That job carried him to a position in the White House. There he lobbied for legislation raising the lifetime cap on mental health to equal that for physical health. He also served as Clinton's spokesperson during the health care reform debate of 1993 to 1994. Then he worked at the State Department.

There are others I could mention—actresses Patty Duke and Carrie Fisher, or TV personality Jane Pauley, for example—but when you and I read about them or Kay Redfield Jamison, or Ted Turner, or Bob Boorstin, we aren't usually told that they have been diagnosed with bipolar disorder. Every time I see a news article in which a killer, or someone who was shot and killed by police, or someone who died by suicide is listed as having bipolar disorder, I remind myself that there are nearly two million of us with bipolar disorder in the United States. That's a lot of people—and very few of them have violent histories.

As for Me: My Life Today

Since my last alcoholic drink and hospitalization around the year 1996, I have much to be thankful for. Treatment has given me another chance at life. *Mind Race* is being published, I have a job, a lovely wife, and a newborn son. I still keep regular appointments with my very talented psychiatrist, and I choose medications, therapy, and bipolar-friendly behaviors (minimizing stress; keeping regular sleep, wake, and meal times; staying social; no drinking or abusing drugs; etc.) to keep my bipolar disorder from flaring up. The hints of mania I still experience from time to time remind me of their previous glory, when I burned twice as bright. But then I stumble and am low on energy and irritable for a few days, and I think of the months or years I spent gray and lifeless when the candle barely burned at all, and I am glad that I have stayed treated. The challenge for me is and will be to keep my already strong marriage healthy, to do my job as well as I can so that it will continue to support my family, to keep my health insurance and deal with rising health care costs, to get insurance companies to pay their bills (document everything and be persistent!), to live with the repercussions of taking long-term medication, and to continue preparing for the possibility of raising a child or children with or without mental disorders.

The hints of mania I still experience from time to time remind me of their previous glory, when I burned twice as bright. But then I stumble and am low on energy and irritable for a few days . . . I am glad that I have stayed treated.

The adventure continues, but partying has been replaced with dinner parties, family time, and keeping our house running. I have a strong family whom I love and who love me, and I don't expect that I will be hospitalized again for my bipolar disorder.

And as For You: Don't Give Up!

You will feel better faster if you leave yourself no other option but to push forward and heal one day at a time. Instead of being bothered by negative comments, such as "just snap out of it" and "why aren't you better by now?" make an effort to spend time with people who are truly supportive. If you believe you can and will get better, you are one step further toward taking charge of your life. If you are able to get appropriate treatment, it is likely your condition will improve. Having a diagnosis of bipolar disorder is not the end of your life, but educating yourself and treating your disorder is the beginning of a new one. Like Jamison, Turner, Boorstin, and others, those in the mind race can be winners, and so can you.

Some Frequently Asked Questions for the Recently Diagnosed

> It was the best of times, it was the worst of times.
> It was the age of wisdom, it was the age of foolishness.
> It was the season of light, it was the season of darkness.
> It was the spring of hope, it was the winter of despair . . .
>
> —Charles Dickens, *A Tale of Two Cities* (1859)

Will I have this illness for the rest of my life?

Yes, bipolar disorder is a lifelong condition, but researchers and doctors are working to find causes and, as a result, possible cures for the disorder, so it is important to stay optimistic about the future. Meanwhile, there are new treatments on the horizon for managing the illness.

If the possibility of a cure seems doubtful, remember that many doubted that Jonas Salk would be able to develop a vaccine to blunt polio. In the early 1990s, who would have imagined that doctors would now be able to significantly delay symptoms of AIDS from occurring in those with HIV infection?

Did I do something to deserve this? Am I to blame for getting it?

NO.

Did my parents do something to inflict this on me? Do I have bipolar disorder because they were bad parents?

Parents don't intentionally cause mental illness in their children. If children are predisposed to having mental illness and they are raised in a dysfunctional family, the genes affecting mental illness may be more likely to express themselves, but ultimately, helping yourself is much more productive than blaming adults.

Are Jerry Springer, the South Park kids, violence in the media, black bile, devils, or over-consumption of soft drinks responsible for the fact that I have bipolar disorder?

Hmmm, probably not.

Why me?

If you'd asked Hippocrates in the fourth century B.C., he probably would have told you that the ordering of the planets elicited black bile from your spleen, producing a dark mood. During the Middle Ages, a diagnostician might have concluded that you were possessed by the devil. Compared with those hypotheses, a combination of a person's genes, brain chemicals, and environment seems to be a pretty benign explanation.

Former president Jimmy Carter once remarked, "Life is unfair." The short answer is that bipolar disorder is treatable and it can affect people of all ages, races, economic levels, etc. The long answer probably includes "luck of the genes" and "historical accident." Historical accident because, according to one theory, a predisposition for depression may exist in one's genes, but it must be triggered by a stressful or traumatic event, such as the death of a sibling or parent, that occurs at a young age. In one incarnation of this view, the traumatic event permanently alters brain chemistry.

For the moment, that is just a theory—but it's an interesting one. The bottom line is that we've had a bit of bad luck. There was roughly a 1% chance of having this disorder, and you and I are in that 1%. If you have this condition, remember that you are not alone and be thankful that there is testing and treatment, that many lead nearly normal lives with this condition, and that unlike many other illnesses, this one doesn't have to be degenerative (become worse over time). Avoiding illegal drugs, seeking stable jobs and relationships, quitting drinking, and maintaining a regular sleep cycle are rewarding experiences, but they're ones that you have to learn to appreciate.

Lots of people have something "wrong" with them or at least perceive that they do. Some people wish they were taller, some feel they're overweight, some say they aren't smart. The important thing to remember is that we're comparatively fortunate. Life bears far worse burdens than depression and mania. Dire poverty and degenerative illness happen all over the world and can be much worse.

In 2004, Richard Cohen, a television news producer, published a memoir titled *Blindsided* about his experience with multiple sclerosis. Because of MS, he has lost much of his eyesight and periodically loses his balance. As a result he has fallen many times, including down the staircase of one of the Manhattan subway stations he uses as he navigates New York City unassisted. He reflects on his life in the following: "I have survived thirty years of a war with my body and countless battles with my psyche. Resignation presides. So does resolve. Personal strength, in the end, wins out. My hope never dies. And, still, I call myself an optimist. I believe that in the end, my life will be better. That is why I can still get up the hill in the heat." If people with more severe problems can deal with adversity, we can live with bipolar disorder.

Can I live a normal life if I have bipolar disorder?

Part of me wants to declare, "Normalcy is overvalued." Another part says, "Normal is in the eye of the beholder." On most days, my life is filled with highly individualistic folk. Their sometimes eccentric behavior is part of their charm.

Another problem with the word *normal* is that it comes into one's lexicon as part of a pair: normal/abnormal. A norm wouldn't be a norm if there weren't deviation from it. Where others use the word *normal* as a synonym for healthy, I prefer the word *typical*. So, I would rephrase a question about normality this way: Can we live our lives to the fullest? Yes. Bipolar disorder is treatable. Learning to manage my disorder effectively took years and multiple medicinal and therapeutic approaches. My health improved even further when I entered the working world and stuck to a regular sleep, work, eating, and social schedule. This is called managing your biorhythms. As long as we are properly diagnosed, maintain a good therapeutic relationship with doctors, have a strong support system, stay professionally treated, avoid and manage stress, keep a regular sleep-wake cycle, and exercise, most of us can spend much of our lives with manageable symptoms.

"Although it is clear that teenagers with Bipolar Disorder are likely to have a variety of problems," writes Jack Lock M.D.,

Ph.D., associate professor of psychiatry at the Lucille Packard Children's Hospital at Stanford University, "their overall prognosis is good. If they continue on medications and get proper assistance with the social and academic problems that may stem from the illness in one way or another, they are likely as a group to do fairly well. Unfortunately, it often takes a number of episodes of depression and mania for them to get real acceptance of their illness and their need for treatment."

If I have bipolar disorder, do I have to take medication for the rest of my life?

According to current medical wisdom, we will always be on medication. The future may hold a cure or therapy that alters our medication requirements, but for now, our best course is to stay on some routine that includes medication and psychotherapy.

The National Institute of Mental Health (NIMH) reports that "With optimal treatment, a bipolar patient can regain approximately seven years of life, 10 years of effective major activity, and nine years of normal health, which otherwise would have been lost due to (manic-depressive) illness also known as bipolar disorder."

What is lithium and what are its side effects?

You may recall memorizing the periodic table when you took chemistry class. If so, you already know lithium not as a wonder drug, but as an element discovered in 1817 and abbreviated as Li. Lithium is the lightest of the alkali metals. It is relatively soft, has a low melting point, and reacts with water.

The lithium we are talking about here isn't actually pure lithium but lithium carbonate. If the thought of ingesting something listed on the periodic table makes you feel robotic, consider that calcium and sodium are also elements. Indeed, our bodies are made up of elements, mainly carbon, hydrogen, and oxygen.

Even though bipolar disorder became treatable with the advent of lithium, which was approved by the Food and Drug Administration in 1970, researchers still have much to learn about this medicine and many others. Lithium appears not to simply treat symptoms but, in medical jargon, to "prophylactically" (preemptively) stabilize "the underlying disease process." Lithium treatments are less effective on subjects who have had more episodes. Also, stopping one's use of lithium can prevent it from working in the future. If you are considering stopping your lithium, remember that you are stopping something that has been scientifically tested and works to control bipolar in many patients. For example, in one study, 37.3% of those on lithium "relapsed," compared to 79.3% of those who were taking a placebo, or sugar pill.

Lithium has several potential side effects, as do all medications. A hand tremor is common, and some people gain weight. Others experience gastrointestinal upsets. Lithium can also reduce thyroid functioning, an effect more common in women than in men. My biggest complaints are having to drink a lot of fluids to overcome a dry mouth and having to urinate more often. Drugs such as valproic acid (Depakote) and carbamazepine (Tegretol) are up to 80% effective in treating lithium non-responders.

A word of caution to lithium users who are also Big Gulp fans and coffee-aholics: A 1995 study reports that lithium blood levels went up 24% in most lithium users who gave up heavy coffee drinking (four to eight cups a day). The researchers warn that those of us on lithium who abruptly stop our caffeine intake are more likely to experience lithium toxicity, something that can happen when there is too much lithium concentrated in your blood. Rather than quitting cold turkey, you can wean yourself off of caffeine gradually. Personally, I drink it in moderation and no later than at lunchtime so I can sleep more easily that night.

I have been told by doctors to drink several liters of water if I feel disoriented from too much lithium. This happened to me once when I accidentally took my medication twice, something I have remedied now by using a series of pill containers that have the times marked clearly with the medication. The study above hints that because caffeine impedes lithium's functioning, it might be good to avoid it. In the process, you will minimize some of lithium's side effects because less lithium will then be needed to achieve a comparable therapeutic blood level.

There are some other concerns about taking lithium. One's lithium blood level can also be dangerously raised by taking NSAIDs (nonsteroidal anti-inflammatory agents) while on lithium. NSAIDs include ibuprofen (some common brand names are Advil, Nuprin, and Motrin). If you are pregnant or planning to get pregnant, you should also know that lithium passes through the placenta and can cause birth defects. It is extremely important to work with your doctor if you plan on becoming or discover that you are pregnant while taking lithium or any other medication.

Because lithium carbonate is a salt, should I decrease my salt intake when I am on lithium?

No! When the level of sodium in the body drops because of diet, heavy sweating, diarrhea, vomiting, or fever, one's lithium level can build up, causing a toxic reaction. When the body loses salt through such activities, the kidneys, which can't distinguish lithium from sodium, stop the loss of salt in urine and in the process stop the discharge of lithium from the system as well. Lithium builds up and can become toxic as a result.

How will I know if I am suffering from lithium toxicity?

Blood levels should be checked regularly as a precaution. According to one source, signs of toxicity include "slurred speech, trouble with coordination and walking, and confusion." If any one or a combination of these occurs, call your doctor right away. And while you're waiting for him or her to call back, drink plenty of water.

I've heard that lithium can cause kidney failure that can kill you. Is that true?

The long-term data suggest that lithium does not "induce renal insufficiency." Lithium can produce negative kidney effects in higher concentrations, however, so drink a lot of water, stay in touch with your doctor, and try not to worry.

Does lithium dull creativity?

The patient is sitting on the examining table, fractured wrist in a cast. The doctor enters. "Doctor, will I be able to play the piano after the cast comes off?" asks the patient. "Depends on whether you could play the piano before it went on," responds the doctor.

If you weren't creative before taking lithium, feel free to use it as an excuse for the fact that you aren't creative now. The research about perceived creativity is counterintuitive. In one study, over half thought that lithium use had increased their creativity! Another quarter thought it had no effect one way or the other.

This question is still being researched. Remember that you will be more productive in most capacities if your illness is being managed and controlled properly.

Will my personality change if I keep taking lithium?

Your core personality will not change. Some artists think being off lithium enhances their creativity (though this isn't a proven phenomenon). The amount of time you spend hypomanic, or having elevated mood or energy but not fully manic, might make you lots of friends, but it is very brief. Most of the time that you are enjoying yourself on an upswing, your real friends are worrying about you. Why worry the people who love you?

Another good thing about taking lithium is that the physical distance between you and whomever you speak to will remain at a comfortable level. When I'm manic or hypomanic, I get very close to people I am talking to, as if I were going to eat their words. Also, lithium levels my moods without confiscating my sense of humor.

How do I know if a medication is right for me?

Talk to your doctor. There are many medications to treat bipolar disorder. All have side effects listed in their packaging that you should read. One approach to avoid feeling too drugged while you are on meds is to work with a doctor who believes in using the minimum effective dose for psychotropic medications, because this helps manage side effects. This also means you have to spend time "tweaking" dosages to find the right blood level to balance your functioning and to keep the side effects tolerable.

There is a huge debate about whether young people should be prescribed "off label"—that is, given prescription drugs that haven't been adequately tested in adolescents and children. Not much long-term data exist on many of these medications in adults and very little exists for children, so there is no simple answer to this concern. Talk to your doctor, keep reading valid health news sources, weigh the known costs and benefits, and always consider whether talk therapies can help you successfully treat and manage your disorder.

What is the relationship between bipolar disorder and substance abuse?

The only way to get a reliable and valid diagnosis of bipolar disorder is first to quit all illegal or abused drugs before being evaluated. Drugs are abused at different levels. I have used alcohol and prescription pills to get to sleep when manic. Many others with bipolar disorder have done the same. One study from 1994 suggested that individuals with bipolar disorder complicated by substance abuse may have more hospitalizations, a higher incidence of dysphoric mania, earlier onset of mood problems, and other psychiatric disorders. In short, self-medication may work in the short term, but only professional help plus appropriate medication can keep us out of the hospital in the long run.

Alcohol is especially problematic. One theory holds that alcohol has a "kindling" effect on the mind. In other words, it helps precipitate bipolar cycling. I have had fewer and weaker bipolar episodes since I stopped drinking. Besides, who wants a beer belly?

Who should I tell about my illness and when?

This is your decision, and no one else's. If you want to keep your condition a secret, don't let anyone bully you into "coming out" about it in the name of fighting the stigma. Yes, a lot of bigots would be surprised by how many of us are in their worlds. And, no, freeing the world of stupidity is not an accomplishable life goal. A strange recommendation from someone who has put his name on a book called *Mind Race*? Actually, it's not so strange. What I would not have done as an adolescent, I am more comfortable doing as an adult. Then again, if the name you see listed on this book as author is Boots Alderwood (my stage name), you'll know that I've wimped out.

I used to tell teens to "tell no one." You don't want to be labeled a freak or give anyone a chance to hurt or shun you because they fear the unfamiliar. Now I say it's okay to tell all of your teachers. If you've got a serious boyfriend or girlfriend, they have a right to know. If they dump you when they find out, they weren't worth the relationship in the first place. More than likely you will elicit the sympathy and support of those who care about you. But I wouldn't announce my illness to a group unless it was a support group.

There are two categories of people in my life: those who know I have a bipolar disorder and everyone else. Teachers are much more understanding if they know about your illness. You shouldn't be put in detention because of illness-related absences. I had an agreement with my teachers (at my private but not my public high school) that I could leave their classrooms and head to the nurse's office at any time without asking. This saved me embarrassment and helped my peers learn without unnecessary disruptions.

Taking time off from work, including vacation time, may be necessary if you are employed and remain hospitalized for more than a few days. What you tell your employer depends on how strong your relationship is. In general you are probably better off with your boss knowing if you think she'll be sympathetic and will limit your travel and unnecessary work stress; otherwise, just say you have a noncontagious illness that's keeping you bedridden. However, during an interview I wouldn't tell a potential employer about my bipolar disorder because many won't "take a chance" on someone with mental illness.

How do you know whether a teenager could have bipolar disorder?

Diagnosing adolescents is a tricky business and must be done by a professional. The Brown University Child and Adolescent Behavior Letter of August 1996 points out that signs of depression in youths and in adults may differ. The letter says, "About five percent of adolescents and 1 to 3 percent of prepubescent children suffer from significant depression."

Signs that someone you know might be hurting from bipolar disorder, according to a 2001 book entitled *Mental Health Information For Teens,* include

Manic symptoms

- Severe mood changes

- Unrealistic highs in self esteem

- Great energy increase; can go with little or no sleep for days without tiring

- Increased talking

- Distractibility

- High risk behavior, such as jumping off a roof and believing no harm will occur to them

Depressive symptoms

- Persistent sadness; frequent crying, depression

- Loss of enjoyment in favorite activities

- Frequent physical illness

- Low energy level

- Major change in eating or sleeping

When diagnosing bipolar disorder, doctors look for broad swings in moods from one extreme to another followed by periods of calm. A study of the components of mania found five factors: (1) a depressed mood; (2) psychomotor acceleration (racing thoughts, pressured speech, disturbed concentration); (3) psychosis (delusions and hallucinations); (4) euphoric mood, humor, increased sexuality, and grandiosity; and (5) paranoia, aggression, and irritability.

What happens during a psychiatric evaluation?

First, make sure that a complete and thorough physical exam has been done to rule out other conditions that produce symptoms similar to those of bipolar disorder. The physical exam will also ensure that your kidney function is normal, an important factor in the decision to use lithium.

The psychiatrist will construct a family history. She will inquire about sleep disorders, drug abuse, physical abuse, neglect, and family conflict. A lot of pain can get churned up and resurface during this process, but remember that you can get better help if the mental health professional knows more about what you've dealt with emotionally and physically. She will also examine the possibility that your symptoms forecast the onset of schizophrenia. Early treatment of an illness is crucial. The Brown University letter notes that "As many as 70 percent of school aged children treated for major depression will have a recurrence of depressive symptoms within a five-year period." Teen suicide is a possibility. This is why warning signs should be evaluated by a professional, just in case.

What modern technological tools do doctors use to evaluate people with bipolar disorder?

Medical technology is useful in treating depression. It can help rule out brain tumors and structural abnormalities. EEGs (electroencephalograms) that monitor brain waves should not be confused with EKGs (electrocardiograms) that monitor the functioning of the heart. An EEG (like an EKG) is painless. Conductive gel is applied to your head and electrodes (small discs) are clipped onto small suction cups that push down on the conductive gel. The cups cover the front, middle, and back of your head. You recline and relax as tiny voltage changes in your brain are detected, amplified, and printed on graph paper. The result is a series of waves that a trained doctor analyzes. The length of an EEG can vary from 20 minutes to a full night of sleep or longer.

The MRI (magnetic resonance imaging) test uses the movement of hydrogen atoms to map the internal structure of whatever it is focused on. It works well on the water-soaked organic tissue of the brain. I had an MRI to rule out the possibility that a brain tumor was causing my depressions.

Recent studies have found structural differences in the brain between those who have bipolar disorder and those who don't. However, these tests at this point are not widely available.

How do I pay for all of this?

Psychiatry is expensive; visits not covered by insurance can cost $300 for 45 minutes. Under most prescription plans, lithium can average around $32 a month. Dosages vary according to a person's body mass and chemistry. Online prescriptions can save a lot of money as well. Being hospitalized for a week can cost thousands of dollars.

If you are among the approximately 40 million Americans who are not insured at all, you have it the worst by far. And if you are insured, you face the bureaucratic soup of receiving convoluted bills. Terry Gilliam's movie *Brazil* highlights the impossibilities of dealing with bureaucracies, and this applies to the health insurance mess in the United States as well. EOBs, or explanation of benefits, are nearly impossibly complicated and confusing and you can be incorrectly charged. People who are desperate, whether they have lots of money or not, sometimes even pay professionals to sort out their medical bills for them. I have spent countless hours on the phone, in personal meetings, and writing letters, and I still curse when I am bombarded by unintelligible bills and am forced to keep fighting to get my treatments covered. In my experience the only way to fix things is to be willing to talk to supervisors, and if you document your phone calls, organize your response to the "assault," and are persistent, you have the best chance of making it work. This broken system hurts the sick, the poor, and the undereducated the most, and it is one of the aspects of dealing with bipolar disorder and managing my health I like the least.

The easiest answer is to be born heir to a fabulous fortune so you can pay for it all with petty cash. Most of us don't have that option. Another is to marry someone who is outrageously wealthy or who at least has access to a family insurance plan. A third is to be adopted by someone who falls into one of the first two categories.

If your parents have health care insurance and you plan to go to college, you are probably covered until you are 23. After that you are entitled to enroll under what is called COBRA for 36 months under your parents' plan. If your parents' plan doesn't cover you and you are admitted to college, you can probably get coverage under a college plan. Most colleges and universities offer them and require that you enroll if you don't have other coverage. If you aren't college bound, your best bet is to get a job with health benefits (unfortunately, something that is easier said than done).

What makes this condition expensive is the fact that many plans cover only 50% of the expenses for so-called mental illness, but (after a deductible) 100% of so-called physical ones. Some states have required parity, which means that mental and physical illnesses are treated in the same way by insurance companies. Most have not.

The second problem you will confront is that unless you have insurance as part of your job after college, you will have to pay a very large premium to stay insured. A law called Kassebaum-Kennedy requires that insurance be available to those with pre-existing conditions (an illness or condition that already exists prior to becoming insured) but does not limit the amount that can be charged in premiums.

The good news is that if you are self-employed, your health insurance is tax deductible. Those who are legally considered disabled by the condition can also qualify for Supplemental Security Income and for Medicaid. To be considered "disabled," you must prove that you are incapacitated to the point that you cannot work. That's the safety net.

By contrast, in 1999, Congress passed the Work Incentives Improvement Act, which allows those with disabilities to work while maintaining their access to Medicare for a period of up to ten years. Those on Medicaid can continue in that program by paying the premiums.

Should I participate in studies about bipolar disorder? If so, what are my rights?

In one of my favorite lines from a Monty Python film, *The Meaning of Life*, an impoverished father announces that his only recourse is to sell off his children for medical experiments. Be fore agreeing to be part of a study, also known as a clinical investigation, you should know your rights. The first is the most important: You can refuse to participate or can end your participation at any time. You are not a guinea pig.

The American Medical Association's Ethical Guidelines for Clinical Investigation state that "the investigator should demonstrate the same concern and caution for the welfare, safety, and comfort of the person involved as is required of a physician who is furnishing medical care to a patient independent of any clinical investigation." Those guidelines also specify that "minors or mentally incompetent persons may be used as subjects in clinical investigation only if: a) The nature of the investigation is such that mentally competent adults would not be suitable subjects. b) Consent, in writing, is given by a legally authorized representative of the subject under circumstances in which informed and prudent adults would reasonably be expected to volunteer themselves or their children as subjects."

Finally, your doctor should not secure your consent by making you think that giving it will result in a better relationship with him. You should not feel or be coerced. The AMA guidelines say that "physicians should not use persuasion to obtain consent which otherwise might not be forthcoming, nor should expectations be encouraged beyond those which the circumstances reasonably and realistically justify."

How can I be a good friend to someone who has bipolar disorder?

My paternal grandmother had diabetes. She had several strokes and relied on her husband for her daily insulin shots. She carefully regulated how much sugar she ate. We treated her differently than we would have if she hadn't had diabetes. We didn't tempt her with sweets and we made sure she ate regular meals. Despite her illness, she lived a full and happy life.

Having a friend with bipolar disorder is similar. Sugar is not the problem. Sleep deprivation, drugs, and stress are. Asking me to go clubbing with you insults me because as a friend you should know that I can't drink alcohol and disrupt my sleep-wake cycle without serious consequences. Offering me a beer is a polite gesture but puts me in an awkward situation. Road trips are great bonding experiences but are also great sources of stress. Now that you know what not to do, how can you be the friend of someone with this illness?

Sometime during my childhood a teacher said that the teachings of the world's great religions can be reduced to two commandments: Do unto others as you would have them do unto you, and love your neighbor as yourself. I want to be the kind of friend who lives up to those two commandments. And, particularly when I'm ill, I want friends to do the same. If an adolescent has a support system that works, it makes the passage through adolescence safer and easier.

Friends who can't accept your illness aren't real friends anyway. Disclosing your illness can also be a way of gaining someone's trust. People often reciprocate and reveal something about themselves when you let your guard down and allow them to be closer to you.

A person with bipolar disorder but without good friends is a person in trouble. As my friend, you are an important resource in my life. When you treat me responsibly, you help me stay healthy. You are my sounding board when I feel episodic tremors. I turn to you when others flee, when I hate myself and am carrying a ton of guilt. When I can't remember the laughs and love, you are there to remind me how funny I am and that what I'm feeling is only temporary. *You remind me that I am not my illness.*

The best thing you can do for friends with bipolar disorder is to be there for them when they are out of control, confrontational, and pushing people away. Besides the countless times you lend a supportive ear, this is when you are needed most. Someone with epilepsy is not responsible for the electrical storm in his brain any more than I am for the harsh words I spit out when I'm manic. You might conclude that we should be able to control ourselves. We can to a degree, but it's harder than you think. Please give your friend some leeway during bipolar episodes. When our minds are pushed to extremes, we say hurtful things we don't mean—especially to those we love.

If it is possible to feel good about being hospitalized, it is most likely that you will feel this way when you are the one making the decision to enter that protected environment. I feel best about the hospitalizations that began with me walking to the hospital with a friend, signing myself in, and spending the time it took to be admitted in my friend's company.

That has happened enough for a pattern to develop. After my friend and I spend a few hours together an argument starts. I want my friend to go home and get some sleep. The clock says that it is past 3:00 A.M. On separate occasions, several of my friends all insisted on staying until I was admitted and medicated. They sat with me on tiled floors and in padded evaluation rooms for hours. Two of my friends made sure I was treated like a human during a dehumanizing process. They fought for my rights when I was too weak to utter a word on my own behalf. Another friend even said he was my brother so he could get past the nurses to visit me after hours.

I wouldn't trade 20 ordinary friends for the kinds of friends I've had during my most difficult times. I feel comfortable telling them things I would feel uneasy revealing to my parents. They are the rope with which my safety net is braided. Having been around me for years and seen me in many different situations, they can judge the difference between manic and happy or between blue and depressed. When the dirt hits the fan (you know what I mean to say), I can rely on them to help me ride out the storm.

Am I protected from discrimination?

Both Section 504 of the Rehabilitation Act of 1973 and the Americans with Disabilities Act of 1990 protect those with mental illness from discrimination. Section 504 bans discrimination on the basis of disability in federally funded programs, activities, or institutions. Section 104.42 of the implementing regulations, according to William Kaplan and Barbara Lee's *The Law of Higher Education* (1995), "prohibits discrimination on the basis of disability in admissions and recruitment" as well as "any pre admission inquiry about whether the applicant has a disability." Kaplan and Lee also note that in *Tanberg v. Weld County Sheriff*, "the federal trial judge ruled that a plaintiff who proves intentional discrimination under Section 504 can be entitled to compensatory damages."

The Americans with Disabilities Act of 1990 states, "No covered entity shall discriminate against a *qualified* individual with a *disability* because of the disability of such individual." An impairment must be medically recognized and must "substantially" limit a major life activity. Mental impairment, a category included under ADA, is defined as "any mental or psychological disorder such as mental retardation, organic brain syndrome, emotional or mental illness, and specific learning disabilities." The ADA applies to educational institutions whether or not they receive federal funds. Title III of the act bans discrimination in places of public accommodation of any sort. Specifically covered by this title are eligibility criteria for services and policies, practices, or procedures among others.

Can I be hospitalized or medicated against my will?

There is a major dispute about how difficult it should be for our families to "commit" us to a psychiatric ward. As a general rule, it is a very difficult process. Some believe it should be easier. Some, harder. There's no right or wrong answer here. Just a lot of frightened people trying to do what's right. If you are involuntarily committed, you are entitled to a court hearing. You can't be medicated against your will unless you pose an immediate danger to yourself or others. This is called crisis medication. The only other circumstances in which you can be forcibly medicated are under court order.

In *O'Connor v. Donaldson* (1975), the Supreme Court decision held that "where a nondangerous patient is involuntarily civilly committed to a state mental hospital, the only constitutionally permissible purpose of confinement is to provide treatment, and that such a patient has a constitutional right to such treatment as will help him to be cured or to improve his mental condition."

In *Lake v. Cameron* (1966), the court held that involuntary commitment was only permitted when alternatives that infringe less on the liberty of the individual are unavailable. This doctrine is known as the "least restrictive alternative" rule.

The writ of habeas corpus is also available to anyone who believes that she is being confined to a hospital illegitimately. This is a judicial process whereby a patient or prison inmate can petition to be brought to court so that it can be determined whether that person has been detained unlawfully and should be released from custody.

What sorts of practical information do I need to know about a hospital?

Here are several questions you and your family should address when considering hospitalization:

- Is your doctor on the staff?

- Does your doctor have admitting privileges at the hospital of your choice?

- Is the hospital accredited by the Joint Commission on Accreditation of Healthcare Organizations (JCAHO)? (This ensures that certain standards of quality are being met.)

- Does it accept your health insurance?

- What are the costs that you will be required to pay?

- Are you being admitted to an open or a locked ward?

- Who is your nurse? Day nurse? Night nurse?

- What are the rules on the ward?

- What are the privileges and how do you obtain them?

- How do you obtain an hourly pass, a day pass, a weekend pass?

- Who is in charge of the ward?

- If you want to sign yourself out AMA (against medical advice), what are the procedures and where are the forms?

Related questions:

- What is the cap on your insurance coverage for mental health care?

- Are you eligible for Medicaid?

- Does your state require that insurers cover mental disorders and physical disorders in the same way?

What should I have with me when entering a hospital?

- An advocate (a family member or friend) who will help you navigate the system and ensure that you are being cared for properly.

- Identification, such as a driver's license.

- Contact information for your referring doctor if you are being referred.

- Contact information of those who should be notified in case of medical emergency.

- No matter how old you are, a copy of your living will could be useful. No, I am not suggesting that hospitalization will prove fatal. Some hospitals want evidence of a living will if you have one at the time of admission. Should an emergency occur, this is a form of protection for you because it specifies the extent to which you want to be sustained on life support systems.

- Proof of insurance coverage (Medicare/Medicaid card if relevant).

- Major credit card if prepayment or deposit is required. Checkbook is an alternative.

- A written list of all of the medications (over-the-counter and prescription) you are taking, including dosages and when you last took each. Bring prescription bottles with you to minimize any confusion.

- A list of all chronic medical problems, including any known allergies. Note any side effects produced by medication in the past.

- A concise one- to two-page history of your illness, including date of onset, dates of past hospitalizations, and family history of mental disorders, if any. Hand this to the resident tasked with taking your medical history.

- Pajamas, toothbrush, toothpaste, comb, deodorant, underwear, socks, at least one set of casual clothes.

Why might I need to consider hospitalization?

Hospitalization is not fun, is very expensive, and is something I will never forget. Indeed, hospitalization should be talked about candidly with your doctor before the need arises, in the hope that you can prevent the need from arising or cope with it if it does. Sometimes it's necessary to readjust medication in an environment in which side effects can be carefully monitored. Sometimes hospitalization is needed because you can't function on your own and require the supervision. Sometimes it is necessary because you are suicidal.

What kinds of restrictions are there in a psychiatric ward?

Like life, psych wards have rules. They're often posted near the entrance of the ward. For example:

> Do not touch other patients. Remember to fill out your meal card each evening. Patients are required to attend community meetings. Lights out at 10 P.M. Visitors must sign in at the nursing station. Visiting hours are 2–4 P.M. and 6–8 P.M. Everything visitors bring into the ward will be inspected.

Somewhere in the white, sterile, structured environment of the psych ward is a primary nurse. The nurse will tell you his or her name and, if you are well enough to permit it, will show you around the floor and explain the rules. But you should also be given a patient's bill of rights. During my stay, they included:

You have the right to be treated with dignity and respect.

You shall retain all civil rights that have not been specifically curtailed by order of the court.

1. *The right of private and unrestricted communication.* Unfortunately, in many of the dozen or so rooms I had during my six hospitalizations, there was no way to call me because the telephone numbers weren't known.

2. *The right to peacefully assemble and form a patient government.* I was elected president of the patient government several times. The group's power was its peer support.

   a. *To be assisted by an advocate of your choice or see a lawyer in private.*

   b. *To make complaints and have your complaints responded to promptly.* I was allowed to complain. Whether my complaint was acted on is a different matter.

   c. *To receive visitors at reasonable hours unless it has been determined that seeing visitors would interfere with your or others' treatment or welfare.* I was allowed visitors. The saddest part was how few people visited the other patients.

   d. *To receive and send mail subject to search in your presence.* Understandably patients who have trouble watching TV can have even more trouble writing letters. It is difficult to focus when on antipsychotic medications.

   e. *To have access to telephones designated for patient use.* At the beginning of five of my six hospitalizations, I was under special observation and had no telephone privileges.

3. *You have the right to practice the religion of your choice or abstain from religious practices.* I brought a Bible with me to the hospital once and a nurse noted my "religiosity" in my medical records.

4. You have the right to keep and use personal possessions as long as it is not contraband and you can sell your personal articles and keep the proceeds.

5. *You may make contracts, marry or obtain a divorce or write a will.* (Hell of a place for a honeymoon!)

6. You have the right to participate in the development and review of your treatment plan.

7. You have the right to receive treatment in the least restrictive setting within the facility necessary to accomplish the treatment goals.

8. *You have the right to be discharged from the facility as soon as you no longer need care and treatment.* This rule sounds like a catch-22—as I mentioned, if you admit you are sick you won't be released, and if you don't admit you are sick, you are "crazy" and need more treatment.

9. You have the right not to be subjected to any harsh or unusual treatment.

10. If you have been involuntarily committed in accordance with civil court proceedings, and you are not receiving treatment, and you are not a danger to yourself or others, and you can survive safely in the community, you have the right to be discharged from the facility. You have the right to be paid for any work you do that benefits the operation and maintenance of the facility in accordance with existing federal wage and hour regulations.

How long would I need to stay in the hospital?

An important thing to remember is that it may take time before you feel better. A good psych ward enforces regular sleep, no illegal drugs, regular taking of medication, time scheduled for therapy, varying amounts of time with doctors, and minimized means of suicide. It may seem like forever but keep in mind that depressions are usually temporary blips on your lifeline. Depression and manias cycle and split but rarely remain stagnant. According to one study in 1999, only 4% of the cases of mania and depression failed to achieve remission after five years. That means there's a 96% chance that your current or future illness can be dealt with. New treatments involving magnetic stimulation, new medicine, and new therapies should give hope to those who are in the unresponsive 4%.

But feeling better and getting the hospital staff to see that you're feeling better can be tricky. In my case, a sign that I am feeling better is when my sense of humor starts to come back as well as my sense of irony. I am getting well. "Not so," thought the resident who asked me about the lunch I had just completed. "So, how's the food today?" he'd asked. "McDonald's reputation is safe," I responded. He wrote something down in his checkbook-sized notepad. Later I learned that he interpreted my response as a sign that my condition was worsening. Were I in charge of the world's psych wards, I'd write above the door: Abandon irony all ye who enter here.

In the psych ward, the independent, creative thinking that is rewarded in the best undergraduate and graduate college courses is confirmation that the patient is unwell. As mental health professionals J. D. Frank and J. B. Frank once noted in their 1991 study of psychotherapy, "Staff members subscribe to an irrefutable conceptual scheme that views any nonconforming behavior as evidence of mental illness and everything they do as therapeutic, even though patients may rightly perceive many of the staff's acts as done for their own convenience, or as punishment for misbehavior." I think a family member meeting with administrators and complaining in writing and in person can remedy injustices, but it is important as a patient to try and retain enough control that that you don't break ward rules.

What can help a patient understand nurses and doctors' behavior is to try to take their point of view when you are balanced and neither manic nor depressed. They have to work in the bleak environment you are complaining about, with some unruly patients and families, they can get injured, their reputation is on the line if anyone gets hurt, and they are outnumbered and want to keep order. But it is difficult to take another's point of view when you are feeling wounded and not thinking clearly. I keep in mind from experience that I will be disciplined if I deviate from the rules, so I behave.

What's involved in a hospital discharge?

It's important to move out of the hospital gradually because adjusting to the outside world is stressful. You do this by getting passes to leave the hospital. A pass is goal-oriented. A friend can take you to a movie. A parent can take you to the dentist. If you are in school, you can be given a pass to go back to a class. Or a pass can simply specify that you can take a group walk with a nurse and other patients. In that scenario, the nurse leading the walks doesn't wear anything identifying him or her so you don't have to worry about people thinking you are on leave from a mental ward.

What does a patient pass look like?

The patient pass itself reveals two things about the hospital system: the perverse effects of the fear of lawsuits and the fact that when all is said and done, in order to stay in operation, a hospital has to be a business preoccupied with ensuring that its doctors, nurses, and janitors are paid. Though they vary from hospital to hospital, most patient passes look something like this:

Patient Pass (for six hours or less)

Patient: Date: Location: Physician:
Purpose of pass:
Instructions to patient:

1. Keep this pass with you at all times.

2. Come back to the hospital on time. THIS IS IMPORTANT FOR YOUR MEDICAL CARE.

3. If you have a medical problem while you are out, call _____.

4. When you come back to the hospital, go to the nurses' station on your floor, and give the nurse this PASS.

I understand the above instructions and agree to follow them. I hereby release the Hospital and my doctors and nurses from any responsibility for me or my medical condition while I am away from the Hospital. I understand that if I do not return to the Hospital on time, insurance coverage for my hospitalization and doctors' fees may be lost. If coverage is lost because I fail to return on time, I agree to pay all hospital charges and doctors' fees for hospitalization.

What can I do to stay well after I leave a hospital?

If after leaving the hospital you act the same way you did prior to hospitalization, or make some of the same harmful decisions (such as not taking your meds) you may relapse. Before you are discharged, make a schedule that specifies activities that will keep you mentally stable. Take your medication. See your therapist. Join a club, get a pet, write poetry, make sculpture, take dance lessons, learn to cook, write a book. (Okay, writing a book might be a bit extreme.)

You haven't focused on the fact that people living with bipolar disorder, and especially those who are untreated, have a higher suicide rate than is typical. Why not?

Portraits of grunge rocker Kurt Cobain, appearing in a number of popular magazines in the years since he killed himself in 1994, seem to glamorize the fact that he took his life. If you are a Nirvana fan, you know that his lyrics reverberate with desolation and death. Unsurprisingly, others in his family suffered from depression as well. He had been diagnosed with bipolar disorder. Was he a martyr to the illness? Should his death be romanticized? Not according to Courtney Love, his rock musician wife and the mother of their child. Love publicly condemned Cobain's decision to take his life.

Media suicide contagion is a problem, especially in young people. In her study of 1,800 media stories about suicide in the United States, Dr. Madelyn Gould, a suicide expert from Columbia University, found that

> a disturbing number glorified and romanticized suicide by implying that there is something noble, heroic or self-sacrificing about the act. Most stories didn't mention mental illness, she said, even though studies consistently show that 90 percent of suicides are committed by people with serious mental disorders such as depression, drug addiction or schizophrenia.

Compounding the problem, there are also plenty of opportunities for young people to see and read about suicides in both popular films and newspapers.

Suicide is taboo in American culture largely because most religions frown on it and it exacts a horrific cost in the lives of the deceased's family and friends. Although feeling suicidal is nothing to be ashamed of, not reaching out for help is. Practice saying "I need help." If you fear the consequences of telling your family, designated liaison, or therapist that you are preoccupied with death, see death as a viable option, or are exploring ways to take that option, then you are in big trouble. When you are not desperate, practice turning to those who love you; it feels good and increases the likelihood that you will seek them out when the world turns desolate and the demons in your head tempt you to seek permanent silence.

Suicide prevention is another good reason to stay on lithium. Researchers Frederick Goodwin and S. Nassir Ghaemi concluded in 1998 that "lithium's effect on preventing suicide is established. A recent review of 22 studies involving more than 150 suicides indicates a 6-fold reduction in suicide with lithium treatment of bipolar disorder compared with no treatment." However, due to methodological limitations in the studies, not all researchers are convinced that lithium has an antisuicide effect.

This isn't a book about suicide prevention, but rather one about getting treatment that works more often than not. People who are suicidal need a mental health professional to work with. If you get treatment, stay on your medication, avoid stress, get enough sleep, and learn optimism, you can avoid a lot of pain and feel better.

When bipolar disorder appears in the news, the story usually recounts a killing or a suicide. We've just discussed one taboo subject, how about the other?

Up to this point, I've focused on how we protect ourselves—from discrimination, from stereotypes, from osteopaths (just wanted to see whether you were still paying attention), from drug reactions, from ourselves. We also need to think about ways to ensure that when manic we don't endanger or threaten others.

At the risk of becoming a bald tire, let me say that the best insurance those around us have that we will not harm them physically is our commitment to avoid street drugs and alcohol. A study conducted for the MacArthur Foundation in 1997 concluded that those with mental disorders who do not abuse such substances as drugs and alcohol are no more likely to become violent than the others living in their neighborhoods. Substance abuse predicts violence among both those discharged from mental hospitals and those in their neighborhoods. The likelihood of violence increases beyond that anticipated from substance abuse alone when combined with a mental disorder that required recent treatment in the hospital.

What are the benefits of staying treated?

Remember that lithium may have an antisuicide effect and that other classes of medications used for the treatment of bipolar disorder appear to help one remain well, that staying in contact with a mental health professional and following his or her advice will help ward off crises, and that you should educate yourself about your treatment options—both the positive and the negative, such as unwanted side effects from the medications. It is best to educate yourself on these topics and discuss them with your mental health professional before starting or stopping medication.

Can a psychiatrist or mental health professional tell when a client poses a risk to himself or others?

The Supreme Court has expressed a lack of confidence in the forecasting ability of psychiatrists and other mental health professionals. In *Addington v. Texas*, according to Robert Levy and Leonard Rubenstein's book *The Rights of People with Mental Disabilities* (1996), the court concluded that "there is a serious question as to whether a state could ever prove beyond a reasonable doubt that an individual is both mentally ill and likely to be dangerous."

There is ample evidence that mental health professionals lack the wherewithal to determine who will and will not prove dangerous to themselves or others. A taskforce of the American Psychological Association concluded as a result that "the validity of psychological prediction of dangerous behavior . . . is . . . so poor that one could oppose their use on the strictly empirical grounds that psychologists are not professionally competent to make such judgments."

"The research indicates that clinicians are better than chance at predicting who will be violent, but they are far from perfect," writes John Monahan, Ph.D., professor at the Institute of Law, Psychiatry and Public Policy at the University of Virginia. "The problem is there is no standard procedure and the field lacks a solid research base for knowing which factors to rely on." In general, psychiatrists and other mental health professionals are likely to overestimate the likelihood that a person will endanger himself or others. One study puts the overestimation of dangerousness at 10 to 100 times the actual likelihood of an instance of dangerous behavior.

Does having bipolar disorder mean that I shouldn't have kids?

No. But it does mean that there is a known heritable condition (unlike all of the unknowns) to factor into the decision. Here are some things to consider. Have you found someone who shares your desire to have a child? Have you considered the pros and cons of adoption? Does your partner understand what having this illness entails for you and would entail were a child to inherit it? Are both of you up to that challenge? Do you have the financial resources to manage it? As I noted earlier, if one parent has bipolar disorder, there is a roughly one in four chance that a child will inherit any mood disorder and a 10% chance that child will inherit bipolar disorder. Bipolar disorder is a mixed bag. Leadership qualities and creativity are associated with it. Those with it may have a few extra watts of brain power that can be harnessed to cope. We've lived with the illness. We know that it is treatable. The treatment for your children will probably be better than it is for us. No one can make this kind of decision for you or for me.

Glossary

What are they saying to me?
What are they saying about me?

Remember vocabulary drills in elementary school? Spell the word. Define the word. Use it in a sentence. Where those words had no necessary relation to each other, the words in this vocabulary drill have one thing in common: They are the terms used by the mental health professionals to discuss bipolar disorder, treatments, and related topics. Think of this section as a glossary for the layperson.

AMA No, this is not the American Medical Association but rather "against medical advice." If you have entered the hospital voluntarily, you can sign yourself out even if those in charge oppose your decision. When you do this, you are leaving AMA. To discourage it, some hospitals specify that they will not readmit you if you sign out AMA. This is a form of institutional blackmail dictated by the belief that doctor knows best. If you didn't believe that, before signing out AMA you might ask yourself what prompted you to sign in in the first place. My advice is when in doubt, don't sign out.

anticonvulsant A medication that helps prevent seizures. Many anticonvulsants have mood-stabilizing effects as well.

antidepressant A medication used to prevent or relieve depression.

antipsychotic A medication used to prevent or relieve psychotic symptoms. Some newer antipsychotics have mood-stabilizing effects as well.

anxiety disorder   Any of several mental disorders that are characterized by extreme or maladaptive feelings of tension, fear, or worry.

attention-deficit hyperactivity disorder (ADHD)   A disorder characterized by a short attention span, excessive activity, or impulsive behavior. The symptoms of the disorder begin early in life and are often confused with those of bipolar disorder.

atypical antipsychotic   One of the newer antipsychotic medications. Some atypical antipsychotics are also used as mood stabilizers.

atypical depression   A form of major depression or dysthymia in which the person is able to cheer up when something good happens, but then sinks back into depression once the positive event has passed.

bipolar I disorder   Full mania plus major depression. At least one manic episode or one mixed episode plus a major depression. Mania must last at least a week. Mania may include hallucinations.

bipolar II disorder   Full depression plus near mania. At least one major depression with at least one hypomanic experience lasting at least four days.

blood level   How much medication is in your blood per some unit of measurement. In other words, are you at a therapeutic dose, have you over- or underdosed, or are you off your meds entirely. Blood levels also determine whether you've been drinking alcohol or taking other drugs—legal or illegal.

catatonic   A state of being awake but not responsive.

chronic depression   A form of major depression in which symptoms are present continuously for at least two years.

comorbidity   When conditions occur together (coexist), such as bipolar disorder and an eating disorder.

conduct disorder   A disorder characterized by a repetitive or persistent pattern of having extreme difficulty following rules or conforming to social norms.

cycling   Transitioning between bipolar mood/energy states—for example, from euthymic (regular) to manic or from manic to depressed or from manic into a mixed state.

cyclothymic disorder (cyclothymia)   Euphoria and depression that alternate but are not as severe as they would be in a major depression or major mania. The condition is chronic and cyclical and must last at least a year in children and adolescents and two years in adults.

delusion   A bizarre belief that is seriously out of touch with reality.

depression   A feeling of being sad, hopeless, or apathetic that lasts for at least a couple of weeks. See **major depression**.

discharge   To release from the hospital. "I am being discharged today" means "I'm getting out of here today."

dopamine   A neurotransmitter that is essential for movement and also influences motivation and perception of reality.

DSM-IV-TR (Diagnostic and Statistical Manual of Mental Disorders, Fourth Edition, Text Revision) A diagnostic manual mental health professionals use to classify mental illness.

dual diagnosis   When a patient's case involves both a psychiatric disorder and drug or alcohol addiction

dysphoric mania   Mania with depression.

dysthymic disorder (dysthymia)   A depressed mood that is less severe and longer lasting than a major depression. The mood lasts longer than two years.

electroconvulsive therapy (ECT)   A treatment that involves delivering a carefully controlled electrical current to the brain, which produces a brief seizure. This is thought to alter some of the electrochemical processes involved in brain functioning.

elopement   Believe it or not, this is the word used to describe a patient who is AWOL or, in more straightforward language, a patient who has escaped from a psychiatric ward.

episode   One bout. An episode can last days, weeks, months, or even years.

euthymic state   A normal mood state—not manic, not depressed.

family therapy   Psychotherapy that brings together several members of a family for therapy sessions.

full remission   No symptoms or signs of the disorder for two or more months.

hallucinations   Hearing, seeing, smelling, or tasting things that others cannot hear, see, smell, or taste.

hospitalization   Inpatient treatment in a facility that provides intensive, specialized care and close, round-the-clock monitoring.

hypomania   A somewhat high, expansive, or irritable mood that lasts for at least four days. The mood is more moderate than with mania, but also clearly different from a person's usual mood when not depressed. Hypomania does not include hallucinations.

informed consent   A person's agreement to participate in a study or to be evaluated for or to receive treatment after being informed of his or her rights as a study participant or a patient. Before participating in any study (while hospitalized or not), read the informed consent form carefully. If you are in a psychiatric ward, have your designated liaison read it as well. Except in an emergency, a doctor cannot treat a minor without obtaining the informed consent of a parent or guardian.

intake   The process you are put through to get admitted to the hospital.

interpersonal therapy (IPT)   A form of psychotherapy that aims to address the interpersonal triggers for mental, emotional, or behavioral symptoms.

kindling   In the nervous system, the tendency to become more responsive with each episode of stress such as that brought on by seizures, mania, depression, or psychosis. The "kindling hypothesis" is a theory stating that repeated episodes of mania or depression may spark long-lasting changes in the brain, making it more sensitive to future stress.

light therapy   A therapeutic regimen of daily exposure to very bright light from an artificial source. Also called phototherapy.

lithium   A mood-stabilizing medication.

locked ward or lock-up ward   In this type of psychiatric ward, the doors to the ward are locked for higher security. Patients who pose a danger to themselves or others are usually put in a locked ward.

major depression   A mood disorder that involves either being depressed or irritable nearly all the time, or losing interest or enjoyment in almost everything. These feelings last for at least two weeks, are associated with several other symptoms, and cause significant distress or impaired functioning.

mania   An overly high or irritable mood that lasts for at least a week or leads to dangerous behavior. Symptoms include grandiose ideas, decreased need for sleep, racing thoughts, risk taking, and increased talking or activity. These symptoms cause marked impairment in functioning or relationships.

manic depression   See **bipolar I disorder, bipolar II disorder.**

Medicaid   A government program, paid for by a combination of federal and state funds, that provides health and mental health care to low-income individuals who meet eligibility criteria.

meds   This term is shorthand for medication. "Have you taken your meds?"

mixed state   Exhibiting symptoms of both mania and depression.

monoamine oxidase inhibitor (MAOI)   An older class of antidepressant.

mood   The dominant way that you feel at a specified time.

mood stabilizer   A medication for bipolar disorder that reduces manic and/or depressive symptoms and helps even out mood swings.

neurotransmitter   A chemical that acts as a messenger within the brain.

occupational therapy (OT)   Exercise or productive work usually organized and supervised by an occupational therapist.

open ward   In this type of psychiatric ward, the doors to the ward are not locked.

oppositional defiant disorder   A disorder characterized by a persistent pattern of unusually frequent defiance, hostility, or lack of cooperation.

pass   Permission to leave the psychiatric ward for some specified period. This is one of the privileges that you earn as part of the process of helping you make the transition back to your regular activities in the non-hospital world.

physical work-up   A physical exam that includes blood and urine checks to assess kidney functioning and medication blood levels.

privileges   In a psychiatric ward, allowances of certain activities. Examples of privileges include a pass, being permitted to smoke, to go on supervised group walks outside the hospital, and to engage in such special activities as art projects.

psychiatric work-up   No jogging shoes required. This is the process of taking a case history.

psychotherapy   The treatment of a mental, emotional, or behavioral disorder through "talk therapy" and other psychological techniques.

psychotic   Having delusions or hallucinations. These can be consistent, congruent, or inconsistent with your mood. Someone who is depressed but thinks he is Nero is experiencing a mood (depressed) incongruent (grandiose thinking) delusion. About two out of three of those with bipolar disorder experience psychotic symptoms at some time. These are usually paranoid (everyone is out to get me) or grandiose delusions (I am the smartest person in the world). During mania, some become psychotic, a word that has entered ordinary conversation as a synonym for someone engaging in "bizarre," unexplained behavior. Although some retrograde groups still do it, it is considered inappropriate to identify people as their symptoms or their illnesses. So, one might say that a person is psychotic if that person is out of touch with reality, but it is inappropriate to say that a person experiencing that state is *a* psychotic.

rapid cycling A person who has four or more episodes a year is said to be cycling rapidly. The episodes can come in any combination of mania, hypomania, mixed state, or depression. Between 5% and 15% of those with the disorder experience rapid cycling. Rapid cycling and mixed states are associated with poorer long-term outcome and with some lack of response to the drugs used to dampen mania.

recurrence A repeat episode of an illness.

relapse The reemergence of symptoms after a period of remission.

remission A return to the level of functioning that existed before an illness.

restraints For a hospitalized patient who is out of control, these devices are used to restrain the patient; examples include bed ties. There are legal limits on the use of restraints in hospitals.

risk factor A characteristic that increases a person's likelihood of developing an illness.

rounds In hospitals, reports by someone in charge to those on the treatment team about individual patients and their progress.

schizoaffective disorder A severe form of mental illness in which an episode of either depression or mania occurs at the same time as symptoms of schizophrenia.

schizophrenia A severe form of mental illness characterized by delusions, hallucinations, or serious disturbances in speech, behavior, or emotion.

seasonal affective disorder (SAD) A form of major depression in which the symptoms start and stop around the same time each year. They begin in the fall or winter and subside in the spring.

selective serotonin reuptake inhibitors (SSRIs) Drugs that increase the amount of the neurotransmitter serotonin and therefore synaptic activity in the brain, which can help heal and prevent depression.

serotonin A neurotransmitter that plays a role in mood and helps regulate sleep, appetite, and sexual drive.

side effect An unintended effect of a drug.

social rhythm therapy A therapeutic technique that focuses on helping people regularize their daily routines.

special observation Close, regular supervision of an individual who hospital staff fear is suicidal or homicidal.

substance abuse The continued use of alcohol or other drugs despite negative consequences, such as dangerous behavior while under the influence or substance-related personal, social, or legal problems.

suicidality   Suicidal thinking or behavior.

switching   The rapid transition from depression to hypomania or mania.

tardive dyskinesia   A serious side effect caused by some antipsychotic medications, especially by the older drugs, such as haloperidol (Haldol), and much less frequently with the newer atypical antipsychotic medications. It is characterized by facial contortions, tongue swirling, and other body muscle movements. This malady is a long-term consequence of medications used for sedation and the treatment of psychotic symptoms that patients may experience when suffering from manic episodes. It's important to remember that tardive dyskinesia usually goes away after the drug precipitating it is withdrawn.

The case   That's you. A case history is a history of your illness or disorder.

transcranial magnetic stimulation (TMS)   An experimental treatment in which a special electromagnet is placed near the scalp, where it can be used to deliver short bursts of energy to stimulate the nerve cells in a specific part of the brain.

tricyclic antidepressant (TCA)   An older class of antidepressant.

unipolar mania   Although not a diagnostic term found in the *DSM-IV*, it is occasionally used to describe those with a bipolar profile who experience only mania and not depression. Also called pure mania.

vagus nerve stimulation (VNS)   An epilepsy treatment that is currently being tested for severe, hard-to-treat depression. It uses a small implanted device to deliver mild electrical pulses to the vagus nerve, which connects to key parts of the brain

ward   Also called a "unit," this is a location for a specific kind of medical treatment or for treatment of a specific class of illness. The psychiatric ward is usually the floor or area of a hospital devoted to the treatment of psychiatric illness.

Resources

Organizations

American Academy of Child and Adolescent Psychiatry
3615 Wisconsin Ave., NW
Washington, DC 20016-3007
(202) 966-7300
www.aacap.org
Referral directory at www.aacap.org/ReferralDirectory/index.htm

American Association of Suicidology
5221 Wisconsin Ave., NW
Washington, DC 20015
(202) 237-2280
www.suicidology.org

American Foundation for Suicide Prevention
120 Wall Street, 22nd Floor
New York, NY 10005
(888) 333-2377
(212) 363-3500
www.afsp.org

Child and Adolescent Bipolar Foundation
1000 Skokie Blvd., Suite 425
Wilmette, IL 60091
(847) 256-8525
www.bpkids.org

Depression and Bipolar Support Alliance (DBSA)
730 N. Franklin Street
Suite 501
Chicago, IL 60610-7224
(800) 826-3632
www.dbsalliance.org
DBSA reports that it is the nation's largest organization that is "patient-directed and illness-specific." A distinguished Scientific Advisory Board guides its efforts. DBSA "educates the public concerning the nature of depressive and bipolar illnesses as treatable medical diseases." DBSA runs a network of support groups, publishes numerous educational materials, and advocates for people with mood disorders.

DBSA has a link on its website at www.dbsalliance.org/Info/findsupport.html that can help you locate the contact information to join a DBSA chapter and support group in the Unites States.

Depression and Related Affective Disorders Association (DRADA)
8201 Greensboro Dr., Suite 300
McLean, VA 22102
(703) 610-9026
www.drada.org
Offers information and support to people with manic depression and depression.

Mental Health Infosource
www.mhsource.com/
Lets you subscribe to list servs for a wide variety of mental and physical health problems and provides new information about mental health in general.

National Alliance on Mental Illness (NAMI)
Colonial Place Three
2107 Wilson Blvd., Suite 300
Arlington, VA 22201-3042
(703) 524-7600
www.naml.org
Has more than 1,000 affiliates helping people with mental illness across the nation.

National Hopeline Network
(800) SUICIDE (1-800-784-2433)
This toll-free 24-hour hotline for people who are seeking help or may be thinking about suicide provides referrals to crisis lines and centers across the country.

National Institute of Mental Health (NIMH)
Office of Communications
6001 Executive Blvd.
Rm. 8184, MSC 9663
Bethesda, MD 20892-9663
(866) 615-6464
www.nimh.nih.gov
This division of the National Institutes of Health seeks to "diminish the burden of mental illness through research." The site offers extensive mental health resources for practitioners, researchers, and the public.

National Mental Health Association (NMHA)
2001 N. Beauregard St., 12th Floor
Alexandria, VA 22311
(703) 684-7722
www.nmha.org
NMHA has a network of more than 340 affiliates nationwide working to improve the mental health of Americans.

U.S. Department of Justice Americans with Disabilities Act
(ADA Home Page)
www.usdoj.gov/crt/ada/adahom1.htm

Books

There is a wide variety of books that deal with bipolar disorder that you should consider reading. Some are written by those with advanced degrees—for example, Frederick Goodwin and Kay Redfield Jamison's *Manic-Depressive Illness* (New York: Oxford University Press, 1990; a second edition is forthcoming in 2007); Peter Whybrow's *A Mood Apart: Depression, Mania, and Other Afflictions of the Self* (New York: Basic Books, 1997); and F. Fuller Torrey and M. B. Knable's *Surviving Manic Depression* (New York: Basic Books, 2002).

Others are autobiographies by adults with the disorder. For example, *Electroboy: A Memoir of Mania* by Andy Behrman (New York: Random House, 2002), is an edgy, engaging memoir of his life in New York City and of his experiences dealing with the complications of bipolar disorder, including treatment with electroconvulsive therapy. Kay Redfield Jamison's *Unquiet Mind: A Memoir of Moods and Madness* (New York: Alfred A. Knopf, 1995) and Patty Duke's *Call Me Anna* (New York: Bantam, 1987) are also highly recommended reading.

Still others are anguished accounts memorializing the lives of those whose illness ended in suicide, such as Danielle Steele's *His Bright Light: The Story of Nick Traina* (New York: Delacourt, 1998); or family guides written by parents and siblings of those with the disorder, such as Diane and Lisa Berger's *We Heard the Angels of Madness* (New York: William Morrow, 1991).

Dr. Martin Seligman's book *Learned Optimism* (New York: Vintage, 2006) is an important book for readers who want to improve on how they think about themselves and the world. And for more information for teens about mental illness, go to www.CopeCareDeal.org, a Web site sponsored specifically for adolescents by the Annenberg Foundation Trust at Sunnylands.

Bibliography

Abrams, Richard. *Electroconvulsive Therapy* (4th ed.). New York: Oxford University Press, 2002.

Alloy, Lauren B., John H. Riskind, and Margaret J. Manos. *Abnormal Psychology.* New York: McGraw-Hill, 2005.

American Academy of Child and Adolescent Psychiatry. "Teen suicide." www.aacap. org/publications/factsfam/suicide.htm. Accessed 9/7/04.

American Academy of Child and Adolescent Psychiatry. "11 questions to ask before psychiatric hospitalization of your child or adolescent." www.aacap.org/ publications/factsfam/11qustin.htm. Accessed 9/28/2004.

American Psychiatric Association. *Diagnostic and Statistical Manual of Mental Disorders* (4th ed.). Washington, DC: American Psychiatric Association, 1994.

American Psychiatric Association. *Desk Reference: Diagnostic Criteria from DSM-IV.* Washington, DC: American Psychiatric Association, 1994.

American Psychiatric Association. *Diagnostic and Statistical Manual of Mental Disorders* (4th ed., text revision). Washington, DC: American Psychiatric Association, 2000.

American Psychological Association. *Report of the Task Force on the Role of Psychology in the Criminal Justice System.* Washington, DC: American Psychological Association, 1978.

Andreasen, Nancy. Creative tension. *Washington Post* (4/16/95), p. W11.

Angst, Felix, Hans H. Stassen, Paula J. Clayton, et al. Mortality of patients with mood disorders: Follow-up over 34–38 years. *Journal of Affective Disorders* 68 (2002): 167–181.

Baldessarini, Ross J., and Leonardo Tondo. Suicide risks and treatments for patients with bipolar disorder. *JAMA* 290:11 (9/17/03): 1517. http://jama.ama-assn.org/ cgi/reprint/290/11/1517. Accessed 8/5/05.

Barbini, Barbara, Francesco Benedetti, Cristina Colombo, Danilo Dotoli, Allessandro Bernasconi, Mara Cigala-Fulgosi, Marcello Florita, and Enrico

Smeraldi. Dark therapy for mania: a pilot study. *Bipolar Disorders* 7 (2005): 98–101.

Basco, Monica Ramirez, and A. John Rush. *Cognitive-Behavioral Therapy for Bipolar Disorder.* New York: Guilford Press, 1996.

Bauer, Mark S. Bipolar disorders. In Allan Tasman, Jerald Kay, and Jeffrey A. Lieberman (eds.): *Psychiatry* (vol. 2). Philadelphia: W.B. Saunders, 1997, pp. 966–989.

Beck, Aaron T., A. John Rush, Brian F. Shaw, and Gary Emery. *Cognitive Therapy of Depression.* New York: Guilford Press, 1979.

Behrman, Andy. *Electroboy: A Memoir of Mania.* New York: Random House, 2002.

Belliner, Karen (ed.). *Mental Health Information for Teens.* Detroit, MI: Omnigraphics, 2001.

Bibb, Porter. *It Ain't as Easy as It Looks.* New York: Crown, 1993.

Biederman, J. Is there a childhood form of bipolar disorder? *Harvard Mental Health Letter,* March 1997.

Brown University Child and Adolescent Behavior Letter, 12:8 (8/96).

Butterfield, Fox. Prisons brim with mentally ill, study finds. *New York Times,* (7/12/99), p. A10.

Carey, Benedict. Talk therapy succeeds in reducing suicide risk. *New York Times,* August 9, 2005, p. F7.

Cassidy, Frederick, Kara Forest, Elizabeth Murry, and Bernard J. Carroll. A factor analysis of the signs and symptoms of mania. *Archives of General Psychiatry* 55 (1998): 27–32.

Centers for Disease Control (CDC). National Center for Health Statistics causes of death 2001 race, sex, age table ages 15–24. www.cdc.gov/nchs/data/dvs/LCWK3_2001.pdf. Accessed 2/2/06.

Chen, Yuan-Who, and Steven C. Dilsaver. Comorbidity of panic disorder in bipolar illness: Evidence from the Epidemiological Catchment Area Survey. *American Journal of Psychiatry* 152 (1995): 280–282.

Cohen, Richard M. *Blindsided: Lifting a Life Above Illness.* New York: Perennial, 2004.

Conlan, Roberta (ed.). *States of Mind: New Discoveries About How Our Brains Make Us Who We Are.* New York: John Wiley and Sons, 1999.

Craighead, W. Edward, David J. Miklowitz, Ellen Frank, Fiona C. Vajk. Psychosocial Treatments for Bipolar Disorder. In Peter E. Nathan and Jack M. Gorman (eds.): *A Guide to Treatments That Work* (2nd ed.). New York: Oxford University Press, 2002, 263–275.

Depression and Bipolar Support Alliance (DBSA). Chapter and Support Group Directory. www.dbsalliance.org/Info/findsupport.html. Accessed 10/18/05.

Depression and Bipolar Support Alliance (DBSA). Bipolar disorder. www.dbsalliance.org/info/bipolar.html. Accessed 10/21/05.

Diamond, Bernard. The psychiatric prediction of dangerousness. *University of Pennsylvania Law Review* 123 (1974): 439–452.

Dunner, David L. Safety and tolerability of emerging pharmacological treatments for bipolar disorder. *Bipolar Disorders* 7 (2005): 307–325.

Emslie, Graham J., Betsy D. Kennard, and Robert A. Kowatch. Affective disorders in children: Diagnosis and management. *Journal of Child Neurology* 10 Supp. 1 (1995): S42–S49.

Endler, Norman S. *Holiday of Darkness: A Psychologist's Personal Journey Out of Depression.* New York: John Wiley and Sons, 1982.

Evans, Dwight L., and Linda Wasmers Andrews. *If Your Adolescent Has Depression or Bipolar Disorder: An Essential Resource for Parents.* New York: Oxford University Press with the Annenberg Foundation Trust at Sunnylands and the Annenberg Public Policy Center at the University of Pennsylvania, 2005

Evans, Dwight L., Edna B. Foa, Raquel E. Gur, Herbert Hendin, Charles P. O'Brien, Martin E. P. Seligman, and B. Timothy Walsh. *Treating and Preventing Adolescent Mental Health Disorders: What We Know and What We Don't Know—A Research Agenda for Improving the Mental Health of Our Youth.* New York: Oxford University Press with the Annenberg Foundation Trust at Sunnylands and the Annenberg Public Policy Center at the University of Pennsylvania, 2005.

Faraone, Stephen V., Joseph Biederman, Douglas Mennin, Janet Wozniac, and Thomas Spencer. Attention-deficit hyperactivity disorder with bipolar disorder: A family subtype? *Journal of the American Academy of Child and Adolescent Psychiatry* 36 (1997): 1378–1387.

Frank, Jerome D., and Julia B. Frank. *Persuasion and Healing: A Comparative Study of Psychotherapy* (3rd ed.). Baltimore: Johns Hopkins University Press, 1991.

Fritz, Gregory K. *The Brown University Child and Adolescent Behavior Letter* 12 (8/96): S1.

Garfinkel, Barry D. Major Affective Disorders in Children and Adolescents. In George Winokur and Paula Clayton (eds.): *The Medical Basis of Psychiatry* (2nd ed.). Philadelphia: W.B. Saunders, 1994, pp. 301–320.

Goodwin, Frederick K., and S. Nassir Ghaemi. Understanding manic-depressive illness. *Archives of General Psychiatry* 55 (1998): 23–25.

Goodwin, Frederick K., and Kay R. Jamison. *Manic-Depressive Illness.* New York: Oxford University Press, 1990.

Gould, Madelyn, Patrick Jamieson, and Daniel Romer. Media contagion and suicide among the young. *The American Behavioral Scientist* 46:9 (5/03): 1269–1284.

Gutheil, Thomas G. *The Psychiatrist in Court: A Survival Guide.* Washington, DC: American Psychiatric Press, 1998.

Gutheil, Thomas G., Forensic Psychiatry. In Harold Kaplan and Bejamin Sadock (eds.): *Comprehensive Textbook of Psychiatry VI* (vol. 2). Baltimore: Williams and Wilkins, 1995.

Hedaya, Robert J. *Understanding Biological Psychiatry.* New York: W.W. Norton, 1996.

Hershman, D. Jablow, and Julian Lieb. *A Brotherhood of Tyrants: Manic Depression and Absolute Power*. New York: Prometheus Books, 1994.

Hollon, Steven, et al. Prevention of relapse following cognitive therapy vs. medications in moderate to severe depression. *Archives of General Psychiatry* 62:4 (4/05): 417–422.

Iqbal, Mohammed M., Tanveer Sohhan, and Syed Z. Mahmud. The effects of lithium, valproic acid, and carbamazepine during pregnancy and lactation. *Clinical Toxicology* 39:4 (2001): 381–392.

Jamison, Kay R. "Manic Depression: A Personal and Professional Perspective," speech given at the University of Melbourne in Australia, July 26, 2000. http://aladdin.unimelb.edu.au/speeches/kjamison26july00.html. Accessed 8/12/05.

Jamison, Kay R. A Magical Orange Grove in a Nightmare: Creativity and Mood Disorders. In R. Conlan (ed.): *States of Mind: New Discoveries About How Our Brains Make Us Who We Are*. New York: John Wiley and Sons, 1999, pp. 53–80.

Jamison, Kay R. February presentation delivered at the Free Library in Philadelphia, PA., 1997.

Jamison, Kay R. *An Unquiet Mind*. New York: Alfred A. Knopf, 1995.

Jamison, Kay R. *Touched With Fire: Manic-Depressive Illness and the Artistic Temperament*. New York: Free Press, 1993.

Janet, Pierre. *La Force et la Faiblesse Psychologiques*. Paris: Maloine in Menninger, 1932.

Janicak, Philip G., and John M. Davis. *Principles and Practice of Psychopharmacotherapy*. Baltimore: Lippincott, Williams and Wilkins, 1993.

Jussim, Lee. In Antony S. R. Manstead and Miles Hewstone, et al. (eds.): *The Blackwell Encyclopedia of Social Psychology*. Oxford, England: Blackwell, 1995.

Kaplan, Harold I., and Benjamin J. Sadock (eds.). *Comprehensive Textbook of Psychiatry VI* (vols.1 and 2). Baltimore: Williams and Wilkins, 1995.

Kaplin, William A., and Barbara A. Lee. *The Law of Higher Education*. San Francisco: Jossey-Bass, 1995.

Karasu, T. Byram. *Wisdom in the Practice of Psychotherapy*. New York: Basic Books, 1992.

Kendler, Kenneth S., Ellen E. Walters, Michael C. Neale, Ronald C. Kessler, Andrew C. Heath, and Lindon J. Eaves. The structure of the genetic and environmental risk factors for six major psychiatric disorders in women. *Archives of General Psychiatry* 52 (1995): 374–383.

Klass, Tim. Study: Cobain suicide failed to spur copycats Authorities feared jump in suicides after rocker took own life. *Peoria Journal Star* (10/20/94), p. C13.

Koocher, Gerald P., John C. Norcross, and Sam S. Hill III (eds.). *Psychologists' Desk Reference*. New York: Oxford University Press, 1998.

Kraepelin, Emil. *Manic Depressive Insanity and Paranoia*. Trans. R. M. Barclay. Edinburgh: E. and S. Livingstone, 1921.

Kruger, Stephanie, et al. Pharmacotherapy of bipolar mixed states. *Bipolar Disorders* 7:3 (6/05): 205–215.

Lamictal home page reporting on FDA release.www.lamictal.com/bipolar/. Accessed 10/25/05.

Lenox, Robert H., and Husseini K. Manji. Lithium. In Alan F. Schatzberg and Charles B. Nemeroff (eds.): *Textbook of Psychopharmacology*. Washington, DC: The American Psychiatric Press, 1998, pp. 379–429.

Levy, Robert M., and Leonard S. Rubenstein. *The Rights of People With Mental Disabilities*. Carbondale, IL: Southern Illinois University Press, 1996.

Lish, Jennifer D., Susan Dime-Meenan, Peter C. Whybrow, R. Arlen Price, and Robert M. Hirschfeld. The National Depressive and Manic-Depressive Association (NDMDA) survey of bipolar members. *Journal of Affective Disorders* 31 (1994): 281–294.

Lock, James. Depression. In Hans Steiner (ed.): *Treating Adolescents*. San Francisco: Jossey-Bass, 1996.

Marshall, Myron H., Charles P. Neumann, and Milton Robinson. Lithium, creativity, and manic-depressive illness: Review and prospectus. *Psychosomatics* 11 (1970): 406–488.

Matson, Johnny L. *Treating Depression in Children and Adolescents*. New York: Pergamon Press, 1989.

Menninger, Karl Augustus. *The Vital Balance: The Life Processes in Mental Health and Illness*. New York: Viking Press, 1963.

Menninger, Karl Augustus. *The Human Mind*. New York: The Literary Guild of America, 1930.

Mental Health: A Report of the Surgeon General. 1999. www.surgeongeneral.gov/library/mentalhealth/chapter1/sec1.html#approach. Accessed 10/18/05.

Mester, Roberto, Paz Toren, Israela Mizrachi, Leo Wolmer, Nathan Karni, and Abraham Weizman. Caffeine withdrawal increases lithium blood levels. *Biological Psychiatry* 37 (1995): 348–350.

Mondimore, Francis Mark. *Depression: The Mood Disease*. Baltimore: Johns Hopkins University Press, 1993.

Mondimore, Francis Mark. *Bipolar Disorder*. Baltimore: Johns Hopkins University Press, 1999.

National Institute of Mental Health. *Bipolar disorder*. NIMH Publication No. 02-3679. 2002.

National Institute of Mental Health. *Depression*. NIMH Publication No. 00-3561. 2000.

National Institute of Mental Health. Bipolar disorder. 2001. www.nimh.nih.gov/publicat/bipolar.cfm#bp6/paras. Accessed 10/17/05 and 10/18/05.

National Mental Health Association. "1996 Campaign Public Opinion Results in: Depression in African Americans Is Not 'Just the Blues.'" www.nmha.org/newsroom/system/news.vw.cfm?do=vw&rid=43. Accessed 10/21/05.

National Mental Health Association. NMHA survey finds many Americans are poorly informed about depression, slow to seek help. *Hospital and Community Psychiatry* 43 (1992): 292–293.

O'Donovan, Claire, Vivek Kusumakar, Gillian R. Graves, and Diane C. Bird. Menstrual abnormalities and polycystic ovary syndrome in women taking Valproate for bipolar mood disorder. *Journal of Clinical Psychiatry* 63:4 (4/02): 322–330.

Painton, Priscilla. The taming of Ted Turner. *Time* (1/6/92): 36.

Papolos, Demitri, and Janice Papolos. *Overcoming Depression* (2nd ed.). New York: Harper, 1997.

Pavela, Gary. *The Dismissal of Students With Mental Disorders*. Asheville, NC: College Administration Publications, 1985.

Penn, David, Abigail Judge, Patrick Jamieson, J. Garczynski, Michael Hennessy, and Daniel Romer. Stigma. In Dwight L. Evans, et al. (eds.): *Treating and Preventing Adolescent Mental Health Disorders: What We Know and What We Don't Know*. New York: Oxford University Press with the Annenberg Foundation Trust at Sunnylands and the Annenberg Public Policy Center at the University of Pennsylvania, 2005.

Plath, Sylvia. *The Unabridged Journals of Sylvia Plath*. Ed. K. V. Kukil. New York: Anchor Books, 2000.

Player, Mack A. *Federal Law of Employment Discrimination*. St. Paul, MN: West, 1999.

Rogers, Carl R. *Client-Centered Therapy*. Boston: Houghton-Mifflin, 1965.

Rosenthal, Elisabeth. Who will turn violent? Hospitals have to guess. *New York Times* (4/7/93), p. C1.

Rosenthal, Norman E. *Winter Blues: Seasonal Affective Disorder: What It Is and How to Overcome It*. New York: Guilford, 1993.

Rosenthal, Robert, and Leonore Jacobson. *Pygmalion in the Classroom: Teacher Expectation and Pupils' Intellectual Development*. New York: Rinehart and Winston, 1968.

Ruehlman, Linda S., Stephen G. West, and Robert J. Pasahow. Depression and evaluative schemata. *Journal of Personality* 53 (1985): 46–92.

Salinger, J. D. *The Catcher in the Rye*. New York: Bantam Books, 1951.

Salmans, Sandra. *Depression: Questions You Have . . . Answers You Need*. Allentown, PA: People's Medical Society, 1995.

Schou, Mogens. Forty years of lithium treatment. *Archives of General Psychiatry* 54 (1997): 9–13.

Schou, Mogens. Artistic productivity and lithium prophylaxis in manic-depressive illness. *British Journal of Psychiatry* 135 (1979): 97–103.

Shackelford, Laurel. New legislation will expand coverage for mental illness. *The Courier-Journal* (10/6/95), p. 2D.

Sonne, Susan C., Kathleen T. Brady, W. Alexander Morton. Substance abuse and bipolar affective disorder. *Journal of Nervous and Mental Disease* 182 (1994): 349–352.

Steadman, Henry J., Edward P. Mulvey, John Monohan, Pamela C. Robbins, Paul S. Appelbaum, Thomas Grisso, et al. Violence by people discharged from acute psychiatric inpatient facilities and by others in the same neighborhoods. *Archives of General Psychiatry* 55 (1998): 393–401.

Strober, Michael, Susan Schmidt-Lackner, Roberta Freeman, Stacy Bower, Carlyn Lampert, and Mark DeAntonio. Recovery and relapse in adolescents with bipolar affective illness: A five-year naturalistic, prospective follow-up. *Journal of the American Academy of Child and Adolescent Psychiatry* (1995): 724–731.

Styron, William. *Darkness Visible: A Memoir of Madness*. New York: Vintage Books, 1990.

Swanson, Jeffrey W., Randy Borum, Marvin S. Swartz, and John Monahan. Psychotic symptoms and disorders and the risk of violent behavior in the community. *Criminal Behavior and Mental Health* 6 (1996): 317–338.

Terman, Michael, Jivan Su Terman, Frederick Quitkin, Patrick McGrath, Jonathan Stewart, and Brian Rafferty. Light therapy for seasonal affective disorder: A review of efficacy. *Neuropsychopharmacology* 2 (1989): 1–22.

Torrey, E. Fuller, and Michael B. Knable. *Surviving Manic Depression: A Manual on Bipolar Disorder for Parents, Families, and Providers*. New York: Basic Books, 2002.

Tumuluru, Rameshwari, Shahnour Yaylayan, Elizabeth B. Weller, and Ronald A. Weller. Affective Psychoses, II: Bipolar Disorder With Psychosis. In F. R. Volkmar (ed.): *Psychosis and Pervasive Developmental Disorders in Childhood and Adolescence*. Washington, DC: American Psychiatric Press, 1996. pp. 57–80.

Wahl, Otto. Quoted in Aaron Levin, Violence and mental illness: Media keep myths alive. *Psychiatric News* 36:9 (2001): para 5. http://pn.psychiatryonline.org /cgi/content/full/36/9/10?maxtoshow=&HITS=10&hits=10& RESULTFORMAT=&fulltext=wahl&searchid-1129665109743_4858&stored_search =&FIRSTINDEX=0&volume=36&issue=9&journalcode=psychnews. Accessed 10/18/05.

Wells, Barbara G., Joseph T. DiPiro, Terry L. Schwinghammer, and Cindy W. Hamilton. *Pharmacotherapy Handbook*. Stamford, CT: Appleton and Lange, 1998.

Winter, Mary. The face of suicide is one worth studying. *Rocky Mountain News* (10/11/03), p. 2E.

Winokur, George, and Paula J. Clayton. *The Medical Basis of Psychiatry* (2nd ed.). Philadelphia: W.B. Saunders, 1994.

Wolinsky, Howard. Roller-coaster extremes; bipolar disorder can be treated. *Chicago Sun-Times* (8/6/95), p. 52.

Yazici, Olcay, Kora Kora, Alp Üçok, Mete Saylan, Özay Özdemir, Emre Kiziltan, and Tuba Özpulat. Unipolar mania: A distinct disorder? *Journal of Affective Disorder* 71:1–3 (2002): 97–103.

Index